P9-DNR-293

WORDS OF THANKS
FROM READERS OF
THE ARTHRITIS CURE

"I thought you should know that your work has revitalized the lifestyle of at least one grateful man. At seventy years of age, I no longer need a cane, and I'm no longer in pain. Last weekend my wife and I danced at a dinner party (I hadn't been able to do that for more than ten years)."

—NORMAN BECK, Peoria, AZ

"Just two weeks, and already the changes are dramatic! Both knees are so much looser, more supple, and stronger. There's less bone-clicking, friction, and pain! Much less stiffness getting out of bed or out of the car—or off my knees in church! I'm ecstatic—and deeply grateful to you!"

—FATHER MILES O'B. REILY of
St. Mark's Catholic Church, Belmont, CA

"I hastened to buy your book and started the treatments as soon as I found the pills. In three weeks my knee had improved immensely and in six it bothered me little to not at all. For the first time in years I am practically pain-free. I need no cane and I need no surgery."

—GEORGE BAKER, El Dorado Springs, MO

"Upon reading . . . THE ARTHRITIS CURE, I began taking [the supplements] as therein prescribed. Within three weeks I noticed improvement. By the time two months had gone by, the osteoarthritis in my knee, elbow, wrists, and upper neck was 98 percent gone! My lower back has improved by at least 65 percent! I have continued to take [the supplements] at a reduced rate to solidify these improvements. Besides this, an added benefit has been a most welcome increase in body and mental energy level."

—ROY FEHER, Tucson, AZ (age 69)

ALSO BY THE AUTHORS

The Arthritis Cure

MAXIMIZING THE ARTHRITIS CURE

A STEP-BY-STEP PROGRAM TO FASTER, STRONGER HEALING DURING ANY STAGE OF THE CURE

**JASON THEODOSAKIS, M.D., M.S., M.P.H.,
BRENDA ADDERLY, M.H.A., AND BARRY FOX, PH.D.**

St. Martin's Paperbacks

NOTE: If you purchased this book without a cover you should be aware that this book is stolen property. It was reported as "unsold and destroyed" to the publisher, and neither the author nor the publisher has received any payment for this "stripped book."

MAXIMIZING THE ARTHRITIS CURE: A STEP-BY-STEP PROGRAM TO FASTER, STRONGER HEALING DURING ANY STAGE OF THE CURE

Copyright © 1998 by Affinity Communications Corporation.

Illustrations on p. 18 and p. 44 © 1997 by Jackie Aher.

All rights reserved. No part of this book may be used or reproduced in any manner whatsoever without written permission except in the case of brief quotations embodied in critical articles or reviews. For information address St. Martin's Press, 175 Fifth Avenue, New York, NY 10010.

ISBN: 0-312-96916-3
EAN: 80312-96916-5

Printed in the United States of America

St. Martin's Press hardcover edition / January 1998
St. Martin's Paperbacks edition / January 1999

St. Martin's Paperbacks are published by St. Martin's Press, 175 Fifth Avenue, New York, NY 10010.

15 14 13 12 11 10 9 8 7 6 5

To my parents, John and Helen, whose love, encouragement, and enthusiasm for learning remain with me always.

—JASON THEODOSAKIS, M.D.

To the millions of arthritis sufferers looking for an answer.

—BRENDA ADDERLY, M.H.A.

Contents

Acknowledgments

To Kate Hamilton for her never-ending energy, love, and support. William Brooks, D.O., my biomechanics mentor whose principles will someday change the face of manipulative medicine. Joseph Valdez, M.D., for his efforts in prolotherapy; and Nga Nguyen, the "Michael Jordan" of reference librarians.
—JASON THEODOSAKIS, M.D.

To Peter Engel, Howard Cohl, and everyone at Affinity for their unending support and encouragement, and to our editor, Heather Jackson, for her strength.
—BRENDA ADDERLY, M.H.A.

An Important Note to the Readers

The material in this book is for informational purposes only. It is not intended to serve as a prescription for you, or to replace the advice of your medical doctor. Please discuss all aspects of the Arthritis Cure with your physician *before* beginning the program. If you have any medical conditions, or are taking any prescription or nonprescription medications, see your physician before beginning the program or altering or discontinuing the use of medications.

Why do we even mention the word "cure" in the same sentence with "a chronic condition"?

Our use of the word *cure* is substantiated by several references. We use the word *cure* to mean the partial or complete relief of symptoms.

Obviously, nothing in the title or content of this book is intended to suggest that the use of the recommended supplements will fully eradicate osteoarthritis. The evidence, carefully collected in this book, substantiates that the nutritional supplements recommended are frequently effective, even for long periods. Even so, we offer no guarantee that *every* individual will benefit from this program.

A Word from
Dr. Theodosakis

I have developed and used the program described in this book with my patients and have seen impressive results. Some of these patients have been unable to get relief from or could not tolerate traditional therapies. Some remain symptom-free— even those who are no longer taking the supplements. As you read this book and decide with your doctor whether to use the supplements, you should keep in mind the following:

- Osteoarthritis is truly a variable condition, that is, two people with the same stage of cartilage damage may have different symptoms and respond differently to treatment.
- If your cartilage is worn down completely to the bone, your chances of cure are remote. However, the program described in this book may still offer you dramatic relief. The program is a safer and perhaps more effective treatment alternative than most standard therapies.
- Some cases of secondary osteoarthritis are reversible, and there are other medical conditions that mimic the symptoms of osteoarthritis. By treating the underlying medical condition, the arthritic symptoms may disappear forever. Therefore, a thorough diagnosis is critical to determine the best treatment.

Foreword

The revolution has begun.

The battle lines have been drawn. In *The Arthritis Cure,* Dr. Theodosakis, Ms. Adderly, and Dr. Fox predicted that the nutritional supplements glucosamine and chondroitin sulfate would cause a revolution in the treatment of arthritis. The prestigious Osteoarthritis Research Society, in its recent consensus statement, has now acknowledged that these long-ignored agents may be beneficial in the treatment of arthritis.

At one time the only article that could be found in a search of the American literature on glucosamine and chondroitin sulfate criticized U.S. physicians for ignoring the rest of the world's vast experience with glucosamine. Now, every major newspaper in the United States has run articles on these supplements. Several television documentaries have revealed their benefits. But, still, the articles in the professional U.S. medical literature are sparse.

I am presently conducting a double-blind, randomized, clinical trial on these nutritional supplements on one hundred people. This is the first such study in the United States. No one knows what the results will be, but it is anticipated that it will confirm the many European studies verifying efficacy for the treatment of the pain of arthritis.

Just two years ago, when I began the first American study on glucosamine and chondroitin sulfate, I never thought I would live to see the day when these events would occur. Why? Because the political forces arrayed against these two substances are *very* strong. You see, the possibility that these nutritional supplements may be effective is a slap in the face to traditional medicine. The agents, labeled as "alternative" medicine, were therefore shunned for many years. Even worse, for reasons explained later in this book, there is absolutely no incentive for drug companies to investigate and then manufacture and sell glucosamine and chondroitin sulfate. They are not considered drugs in the United States, but simply nutritional supplements, and drug companies can make no health claims for them, however truthful those claims are. Therefore, from a business point of view, there is no point in spending money on advertising. On the other hand, millions upon millions are spent advertising NSAIDs (non-steroidal anti-inflammatories). Most people think of these drugs as being helpful and benign. And, used properly, for the most part they are. But for those who are forced by pain to depend on them, increasing the dosage and frequency in order to combat their worsening pain, the side effects can be genuinely tragic. My grandfather, a pharmacist, died from the side effects of aspirin. But chondroitin and glucosamine have no known side effects.

The battle is intensifying because the effectiveness of those agents can now be further enhanced, as you will read in this book. The result is that, before too much longer, osteoarthritis will be generally recognized as a medically treatable, and possibly even preventable disease.

The next frontier lies in the treatment of rheumatoid arthritis. Already, important advances are being made. Early indications suggest that glucosamine-chondroitin may be helpful for rheumatoid as well as osteoarthritis. Type II collagen offers substantial new hope. Hyaluronic acid, an injectable agent with a chemical composition that has striking similarities to chondroitin sulfate and glucosamine, which has recently been approved by the Food and Drug Administration (FDA), may prove to be useful as well. And there is more to come. This scourge, too, is starting to retreat under the assault of "alternative" medicine. Traditional and alternative medicine will blend, incorporating the best of both; then, finally, the battle will truly be won.

—AMAL K. DAS, JR., M.D.

An Introduction to the Maximizing Plan

About thirty-five million Americans suffer from osteoarthritis. Until the astonishing solution offered in *The Arthritis Cure* was introduced to the lay public, these sufferers (and most of their doctors) believed that the constant ache, the sometimes excruciating pain, and the steadily rising lack of mobility associated with osteoarthritis were the inevitable side effects of aging.

A visit to the doctor would rarely yield positive results. Usually, patients would leave with a prescription for painkillers and the admonition to learn to "live with" their increasingly debilitating condition. But what kind of life is one filled with pain—and with the knowledge that it will inevitably worsen?

The Arthritis Cure Works: New Evidence

Fortunately, as explained in *The Arthritis Cure,* osteoarthritis symptoms can be relieved, halted, reversed, and in many cases cured by following a program that includes taking glucosamine and chondroitin sulfates as the cornerstone of a nine-part plan. These supplements, which increase the body's ability to regenerate healthy cartilage, have been found to be highly beneficial and without unpleasant or dangerous side effects.

The Arthritis Cure has changed the lives of many osteoarthritis sufferers. No longer are they prisoners of a disease that limits their mobility and harms their lives. Indeed, their mobility has increased, their pain has been reduced—and their optimism levels are soaring!

This latter point is very important. Not all the symptoms of osteoarthritis will be eliminated for all sufferers. Yet the fact that something *can* be done, that this is not a hopeless condition, has a wonderfully energizing impact. Glucosamine and chondroitin, in conjunction with the rest of our program, actually alleviate the condition for many and offer hope for many more. But even for those whose symptoms are so severe that glucosamine and chondroitin can make only a slight improvement, the program "bucks them up," energizing them and giving them new spirit. They do more, eat better, and live more completely. And the added exercise, improved nutrition, and heightened zest for living further help minimize the effects of the disease.

Of course, there are always pessimists and naysayers among us. As a result, inevitably some critics have complained that the efficacy of the program has not yet been adequately proved. They maintain that, while some people do report improvement, it's too early to report a full cure. In other words, they are telling sufferers not to utilize a program that might well work for them *because there is not enough evidence to prove that it* always *works for* everyone. In the past, we found that argument to be specious on its face. Now, however, it has been rated completely invalid. There is a lot more evidence—from both the experiences of patients who have used the cure successfully and sophisticated new research studies—that the program really does work.

New Information, New Supplements

There is more good news.

Because of the dramatically increased interest in osteoarthritis stemming from the fact that we were able to inform both osteoarthritis sufferers and physicians about the benefits of glucosamine and chondroitin, a lot of additional research on osteoarthritis has been done or is now underway. Part of this research strengthens our earlier conclusion that those supplements are truly effective; while other research has concentrated on finding new ways to make them even more effective. As a result, several new supplements that will enhance the effectiveness of glucosamine/chondroitin are now either on the market or being readied for sale. (We discuss these in detail in Chapter 7.) Since not all of these approaches are yet fully researched, in some cases we may again be accused of prematurely announcing advances. But, in this respect, you can be sure of two things: We recommend only supplements that are entirely safe; and we clearly differentiate between new supplements we *believe* will improve the effectiveness of glucosamine and chondroitin although more research is needed to be positive, and those where the research already proves the point beyond reasonable doubt. With these informational tools at hand, you can decide for yourself what is best for you.

Our view is that if a product that has a good chance of helping you, can replace a treatment or drug that has known potential to *harm* you, and it has no known negative side effects, why not try it?

Maximizing the Arthritis Cure

Millions of people are now using the chondroitin and glucosamine combination and following the nine-step cure we proposed in *The Arthritis Cure*. Many of them report that the program has essentially cured them. They are playing tennis again or romping with their grandchildren, with a vigor they haven't been able to manage in years. Others report only partial improvement, and it is both to them and to the skeptics and naysayers who have yet to try our approach to curing osteoarthritis that this book is addressed. Once we prove the skeptics wrong by dint of some very impressive research, our main goal is to show you how to maximize the effectiveness of the cure.

You will find in these pages a step-by-step plan for faster, more complete, more effective healing that starts with the nine-point program we outlined in *The Arthritis Cure.* But it also incorporates several new findings and provides you with a more complete program for further implementing and tailoring the cure to your unique problems and lifestyle.

Working with Your Physician

To get the most out of this program, we believe strongly that you should incorporate it into an overall, physician-supervised health plan. Now that most doctors accept glucosamine and chondroitin as an effective treatment for osteoarthritis, this integrative process is much easier for you to arrange. In Chapter 3, we give you a detailed plan on how to work most efficiently and effectively with your physician and/or any other health care professional whose help you need.

An Eating Program Tailored to Your Specific Needs and Tastes

As we discuss in Chapter 6, diet and nutrition are of vital importance to the successful treatment of osteoarthritis—and for assisting in controlling the symptoms of rheumatoid arthritis—in two ways.

• More information is becoming available about minerals, trace minerals, antioxidants, and other supplements that help your overall health and may be of specific value in dealing with osteoarthritis. While these supplements are often widely available in pill, capsule, or tablet form, many practitioners feel that it is better to obtain as many of them as possible from your natural food intake, using manufactured "supplements" only to make good any shortfalls your menu leaves open. Therefore, we show you how to incorporate the foods most rich in these nutrients into your diet.

• Weight control is vital for controlling the symptoms of arthritis. Clearly, if you place more pressure on certain joints than they and the muscles surrounding them were intended to handle, they will wear out faster and hurt more. That is not to say that trying to be as thin as a rail is necessarily a good idea. On the contrary, maintaining a sensible weight for your gender, body size, and age is the best way to deal with arthritis symptoms and with healthy living in general. To that end, we provide you with examples and directions on how to eat appropriately (in conjunction with the exercise program we describe later) to achieve and maintain the weight you need.

Nutritional Supplementation

As noted, not all of the nutrients you need are available in your diet. So we provide you with a detailed program of what other supplements you need to take, how they work, and why they're important to maximizing your arthritis cure.

Biomechanics Exercises

Simply put, biomechanics involves learning to lie, sit, stand, and move in a balanced way so that any shock or weight your body has to bear is distributed evenly across its widest possible expanse. In that way, no single bone or joint has to carry more than its fair share of the load.

An Exercise Program

This part of the program shows you how to increase your strength, especially the strength of muscles that protect your arthritis "hot spots." (Hot spots are meant in a lay sense, and do not refer to the problems of rheumatoid arthritis.) For example, if the joints of your knees are sore, you need to exercise them in order to increase the flow of healing, lubricating synovial fluid to the cartilage. But you also need to protect them from excessive jarring and weight, and that can be done by improving the strength and resilience of the muscles surrounding them.

At the same time, you need to improve your aerobic capacity. This is important for your general health in any case, but it is especially important for arthritis sufferers because aerobic exercise (in conjunction with an appropriate eating program, of course) helps you maintain your optimum weight, increases general mobility, and adds to your energy. That extra energy helps fuel more productivity and makes exercise more enjoyable. And if you are overweight, it also makes weight loss far easier, which gives you a further boost in energy. All in all, a very positive upward spiral!

Naturally, everyone's capacity for exercise varies, as do the "hot spots" for any particular case of arthritis. Thus, we give you a program of exercise designed to allow you to tailor the program to fit your specific needs.

The Toughest Arthritis Problems

Unfortunately, not all types of arthritis will respond to conservative care. Very advanced cases of osteoarthritis, where there is virtually no cartilage left or where not only the cartilage but also the bone itself has been damaged, may be helped but cannot be effectively overcome by chondroitin and glucosamine. Had sufferers of such advanced conditions known about these supplements when their symptoms first began, they might have been able to avoid all or many of their current problems. But since they couldn't have known, now they may have to face a very different situation.

Here again, however, there is good news: There are new ways of dealing with such advanced conditions, ranging from a form of injection to some very clever surgical techniques. We describe these in Chapter 10 and emphasize that injections or surgery should be performed only after an extensive trial of conservative measures, including the entire *Arthritis Cure* treatment program. Thereafter, in the large majority of cases, the benefits of glucosamine and chondroitin and the maximizing program should prevent any further surgery from becoming necessary.

Hope for Rheumatoid Arthritis Sufferers

Rheumatoid arthritis (RA) presents another serious and intractable problem. RA is a different disease from osteoarthritis. Rather than resulting from the *wearing down* of cartilage, it involves the *inflammation* of the cartilage and the consequent swelling of the joints. As we discuss in Chapter 8, this condition cannot yet be cured by chondroitin and glucosamine or by anything else. However, here again, there is good news on two fronts.

The first is that sometimes people suffering from rheumatoid arthritis are also suffering from osteoarthritis. The arthritis cure, in dealing with the latter, will greatly ease the discomfort of the sufferer. It is bad enough that joints with worn cartilage from osteoarthritis grind and ache; it is that much worse if they are also inflamed and swollen. Glucosamine and chondroitin do help with inflammation and by allowing the eroded cartilage to heal, can only help the overall situation.

Second, there are reports that glucosamine and chondroitin have been working in some RA patients. Further, some promising supplements, such as enzyme mixtures and various anti-inflammatory oils, may have a salutary effect on rheumatoid arthritis. Such supplements, these early studies suggest, not only reduce inflammation of the joints—which helps with the pain of RA—but may actually have positive long-term effects. We therefore believe that eventually, rheumatoid arthritis, like osteoarthritis, will be alleviated by or put into remission through the use of these natural supplements. In Chapter 8, we provide you with up-to-date research as well as discuss which supplements promise the most.

In Summary

Maximizing the Arthritis Cure allows you to take another important step forward. This book helps you in four ways.

- It provides you with the reassurance that the glucosamine/chondroitin combination really *does* work. Even the skeptics now agree.
- It reveals new breakthroughs that make these two basic supplements work even more effectively.
- It shows you, step by step, how you can eat, exercise, and improve your body's biochemics so that glucosamine/chondroitin and its various enhancements can become an even more effective treatment.
- It gives you solid information about what you can do if your osteoarthritis has gone too far to be fully treatable with the recommended supplements. If you suffer from rheumatoid arthritis, it provides you with information on new methods that may help alleviate RA.

If you follow the precepts laid down in this book—and they are not hard to follow, especially when compared to how hard it is to live with osteoarthritis—you will find yourself living a healthier, freer, more productive, and vastly happier life.

The Arthritis Cure Revisited and Improved

Osteoarthritis is a complicated condition but one that can be successfully treated by the application of the program presented in this book. In this chapter, we give you an overview of what that cure entails. In the process, we describe what arthritis is, recap the benefits of glucosamine/chondroitin, and summarize the five parts of the cure. In later chapters, we provide you with details about each of the parts.

What Is Arthritis?

Arthritis is the "sword" jabbing into your knee, the "vise grip" squeezing mercilessly on your shoulder, the "super glue" holding your fingers in contorted and useless configurations, the "ton of pressure" bearing down on your spine. It's one of the major reasons that people go to their doctors, and it is the number-one cause of disability.

So prevalent is the disease that it can be called an epidemic.

- It afflicts nearly forty million Americans, about one in seven people in this country.
- Without a cure, by the year 2020, that number would grow

to more than fifty-nine million based on the demographics of an aging population.
- Some seven million of us have difficulties with living a normal life because of arthritis.
- The total cost for the disease, including medical care and lost wages, comes to just under *$65 billion* a year in the United States alone.

Arthritis is a cruel condition, striking young people as well as old. One form of the disease, called juvenile arthritis, "specializes" in attacking children. Overall, however, arthritis tends to be an affliction of the middle-aged and elderly. Less than 1 percent of those under the age of seventeen suffer from it; 29 percent of those between the ages of forty-five and sixty-four are afflicted; and almost half of those sixty-five and older have "documented" arthritis. We don't know how many more sufferers with painful joints have never been properly examined and diagnosed. This group undoubtedly includes many senior citizens who, believing the condition to be just another incurable manifestation of old age, take some analgesics, rub their aching joints, and never bother to seek professional help.

Arthritis strikes both men and women, although women are somewhat more likely than men to suffer from the disease. Some forms of arthritis, such as rheumatoid arthritis, fibromyalgia, and lupus, are more prevalent among women. Others, including gout and an arthritis of the spine called ankylosing spondylitis, are more common in men. Children suffering from juvenile arthritis form only a very small percentage of sufferers, but they constitute what is obviously a particularly poignant group.

Arthritis Comes in Many Guises

Arthritis is a general term used to describe a group of more than one hundred diseases that strike the joints. Some forms, such as osteoarthritis, remain confined to the joints. Others, including lupus, spread beyond, attacking the skin, many internal organs, and even the blood and circulatory systems.

Rheumatoid arthritis (abbreviated RA) is an autoimmune disorder that afflicts the entire body. When someone is suffering from an autoimmune problem, instead of protecting the body from disease, the immune system attacks the body's tissues or cells. With RA, this "attack" is particularly fierce on the joints. No one knows why RA develops, although a virus or other infection may be the triggering factor. Symptoms of RA include joint pain, swelling, tenderness, and stiffness. The disease tends to be symmetrical, attacking the same joints on separate sides of the body (for example, both knees or both wrists). General fatigue and persistent aching are also common symptoms, along with muscle pain, loss of appetite and weight, fever, and the development of small nodules under the skin. Less common but potentially dangerous symptoms of RA include problems with the heart and lungs.

Juvenile rheumatoid arthritis can be mild or severe. Depending on the form it takes, it can cause joint inflammation, fever, rash, and damage to internal organs, with symptoms varying from day to day or even from morning to evening. The causes of the disease are unknown, although an inherited genetic trait is believed to play a role.

Lupus, more properly known as systemic lupus erythematosus, is also an autoimmune system disease. For unknown reasons, the immune system turns on the victim and attacks various body parts, including the heart, circulatory and nervous systems, kidneys, and skin.

Gout, which primarily attacks men, is brought about by excess amounts of uric acid in the blood (due either to overproduction, underexcretion, or a combination of both). The uric acid crystallizes and settles in the joints and other body tissues, causing sudden and severe pain, tenderness, swelling, redness, and warmth in the joints, especially those of the big toe and knee.

Anklylosing spondylitis causes vertebrae to fuse together, making the once-flexible spine rigid. Usually striking young men between the ages of sixteen and thirty-five, it begins with stiffness and pain in the lower back and hips. For unknown reasons, this disease is three times more common in whites than in blacks, running in families and apparently having an important hereditary component.

Osteoarthritis is by far the most common of all the many forms of arthritis. Generally striking in the fourth decade of life and onward, osteoarthritis afflicts close to 35 million Americans. The disease causes joint tissue to break down, resulting in pain, stiffness, and, less frequently, swelling. Any joint can fall prey to this form of arthritis, but the most common are the knees, hips, fingers, feet, and spine.

As illustrated by the preceding examples of only six types of arthritis, the disease comes in many guises and is difficult to describe in just a few words. It can strike all ages and both sexes. It may cause just a small amount of damage to a single joint; it may immobilize a once-supple spine; or it may incite the body's defender, the immune system, to run amok. Symptoms of the numerous forms of arthritis range from occasional mild pain to extreme fatigue, from weight loss to heart trouble, from mild annoyance to complete disability. Symptoms may be stable for years, or they may fluctuate wildly. Some forms of the disease are caused by injury; others, we believe, are due to genetic errors; yet still others may be the result of environmental factors including what we eat or fail to eat.

There's a lot we don't understand about arthritis. This much, however, we do know: Osteoarthritis, the most common form of the disease, can now be successfully treated. It is not an inevitable symptom of aging, and it does not always have to worsen with the passage of time. Eroded or damaged cartilage *can* be repaired. As it turns out, osteoarthritis is *correlated* with age, not *caused* by it. That new perspective means that it should no longer be viewed as inevitable. It can be stopped. There is hope.

Osteoarthritis

Osteoarthritis affects the cartilage, the tissue that cushions the joints. The word *osteoarthritis* literally means "bone/joint inflammation," although, in fact, inflammation is not a problem for most people with the disease. The most significant symptom is pain, which can range from mild to debilitating. That pain arises because the cartilage, which in healthy joints separates and protects bone ends so that they glide smoothly and easily over each other, can no longer do its job.

Cartilage is a rubbery, gel-like tissue that sits on the ends of bones, like a cap sits on your head. Composed of about two-thirds water, it is designed to reduce friction and blunt the force of bone ramming into bone as we move about. Properly "irrigated," the watery cartilage, soaking with the slippery synovial "lubricating" fluid, also aids bones by providing the ends with a smooth surface. Five times slicker than ice, cartilage allows bone ends to move easily through their ranges of motion without "sticking" on rough spots.

Imagine filling a sponge with water, then slowly compressing it with your hand. The water seeps out of the sponge as you apply pressure, then gets sucked back in when you release your hand. Healthy cartilage behaves much like that sponge, alternately "drinking in" the synovial fluid that bathes joints, then letting it slowly seep out.

When there is no pressure on a joint, fluid flows into the cartilage, bringing with it the various nutrients needed to keep cartilage strong and healthy. Then, when pressure is exerted, the fluid seeps out of the cartilage, absorbing and dispersing the pressure's force. For example, when you step onto your right leg, the pressure of your weight forces synovial fluid out of your right knee joint. Meanwhile, however, the pressure is off your left knee, so the cartilage in that joint quickly fills with nourishing, cushioning fluid. As soon as you step onto your left leg, the situation is reversed. Rapidly flowing in and out in response to the pressures created by walking, lifting, jumping, dancing, running, and otherwise moving about, fluid fills then drains from healthy cartilage, protecting bones by absorbing shock and preventing them from slamming into each other.

Exercise Is Essential

This mechanism for "sponging up" liquid into the cartilage is why exercise—which may seem to be a paradoxical therapy for arthritis and may even seem dangerous—is not only safe but also essential for arthritis sufferers. *Not* exercising is harmful; regular exercise works like a medicine for damaged joints. Just as with muscles, we have to "use or lose" our joints. And it is only by exercising that we can stimulate the flow of synovial fluid in and out of the cartilage. Since there is no automatic pumping mechanism for the fluid that nourishes the cartilage (like the system the heart has for pumping blood through the cardiovascular system), without the stimulation of these fluids through exercise our cartilage would slowly dry out.

Exercise not only helps keep joints healthy by assisting the flow of synovial fluid, it also strengthens the muscles, tendons, and supporting joints. Strong and well toned, these supporting structures also can protect joints by absorbing much of the force that assaults them as we move.

Under ideal conditions, cartilage would last a lifetime, possibly showing a few signs of age-related wear and tear in our later years but continuing to perform well. Unfortunately, conditions in real life are rarely ideal. We're subjected to minor inherited misaligned joints, various accidents and trauma, and poor nutrition, obesity, and other factors that put excessive strain on our joints. When that happens, cartilage can begin to break down.

Osteoarthritis may begin with a little tear in the cartilage, perhaps due to an injury, the clogging of a blood vessel to the joint, obesity, or poor joint alignment. The body immediately attempts to repair the problem, but sometimes the new cartilage laid down is of inferior quality. Or perhaps there was no initial injury, and the cartilage began to break down because the chondrocyte, the birthplace of new cartilage, no longer functions properly due to age, poor nutrition, infection, or some form of damage. Whatever the cause, in osteoarthritis the cartilage does not function as intended. It begins to break down and no longer fills completely with fluid when the pressure is removed from a joint. Unable properly to absorb and disperse pressure, some of the pressure impacts excessively on the bones, damaging them. That damage, of course, exacerbates the problem so that the cartilage continues to degenerate. Eventually, it no longer acts as a slippery surface for the bone ends to slide across, causing the full symptoms of osteoarthritis.

Pain is the inevitable symptom of osteoarthritic joints. Other possible problems include joint crackling (crepitus), a reduction in the range of joint movement, abnormal hardening of the bones (eburnation), bone spurs (osteophytes), fluid-filled pockets (subchondral cysts), inflammation, bone deformity, joint enlargement, and general immobility. In some cases the cartilage disappears entirely, so that the exposed and unprotected bone ends within the joint rub against each other with every movement. (In the past, surgeons removed the cartilage as part of the treatment for joint problems. We now know that this was *not* an effective approach.)

Traditional Treatments for Osteoarthritis

Doctors generally prescribe acetaminophen and/or nonsteroidal anti-inflammatory drugs for treating osteoarthritis.

Acetaminophen is sold without a prescription under names such as Tylenol, Liquiprin, and Datril. The nonsteroidal anti-inflammatory drugs, called NSAIDs (pronounced ''n-sayds''), are sold over the counter as aspirin, Motrin, Orudis, Advil, Aleve, and other familiar names. They're also available in prescription strength as Indocin, Feldene, Naprosyn, Daypro, and Relafen, among others. Both acetaminophen and NSAIDs relieve pain and reduce fever. However, only NSAIDs reduce inflammation.

Both acetaminophen and NSAIDs effectively reduce pain in many cases, but their benefits come with strings attached. *All* drugs have side effects. For example, in standard doses of up to 4 grams per day, acetaminophen is safe for most people when taken for short periods of time. Unfortunately, millions of arthritis sufferers take acetaminophen or other medications for months or years at a time, which can cause a small yet significant decline in liver function and can damage the kidneys. Indeed, long-term heavy use of acetaminophen-related products is felt to be responsible for up to five thousand cases of kidney failure every year in the United States.[1] This number is expected to increase due to a push of using acetaminophen over NSAIDs in hip and knee osteoarthritis, as recommended by the American College of Rheumatology in 1995.[2]

Aspirin and the other NSAIDs can be even more damaging. While occasional use or continued use in small quantities is rarely harmful, it is of little value in dealing with the continuing, severe pain of osteoarthritis. Nevertheless, to try and counteract that condition, patients often feel forced to take substantial quantities daily. Such usage can have quite nasty side effects, including dizziness; nausea; depression; drowsiness; swelling of the feet, face, or legs; constipation; diarrhea; insomnia; ringing in the ears; dry mouth; tremors; tingling or numbness in the feet or hands; rapid weight gain; ulcers in the mouth; confusion; rashes; convulsions; blurred vision; black or bloody stools; rapid heartbeat; chest tightness; bloody urine; excessive bruising; unusual bleeding; jaundice; fainting; abdominal pain; weakness and fatigue. Some of these side effects, including dizziness and nausea, are relatively common, while others, such as convulsions and bloody urine, are rare. Common or rare, they point to the tremendous potential for damage faced by the tens of millions of Americans taking NSAIDs regularly for osteoarthritis. It has been estimated that there are more than 75,000 hospitalizations and 7,500 deaths each year directly attributable to NSAID use in the United

1. D. P. Sandler, "Analgesic Use and Chronic Renal Disease," *The New England Journal of Medicine* 320 (1989): 1238–43.
2. *Arthritis and Rheumatism* 38, no. 11 (November 1995): 1535–40.

States.[3] NSAIDs are the number-one cause of reported drug interactions every year.

On the positive side, acetaminophen and the NSAIDs can be helpful, especially with short-term pain. But at best they only mask the symptoms, doing nothing to cure the underlying problem, which is the degeneration of the cartilage matrix and the breakdown of joint function. In fact, a new body of growing evidence suggests that some NSAIDs may actually *worsen* osteoarthritis by interfering with the production of the proteoglycans, which attract and hold the fluid so essential to cartilage.

The sad truth is that until recently doctors had very little to offer osteoarthritis patients. There were pills to ease the pain and mask the problem, but they did nothing to solve it and might even have made the arthritis worse. Surgery was painful and at best only partially effective, and physical therapy reduced pain and improved mobility only to a limited extent and only in some cases. Various devices (such as special can openers) help patients get through the day, but there was no cure for osteoarthritis. Until now.

The New Treatment—The Arthritis Cure

With your mind's eye, picture a thin sheet of cartilage. It looks like a piece of paper. As you zoom in for a closer view (Figure 1), you notice that the cartilage structure is composed of what appears to be netting, the vertical fibers interwoven with their horizontal counterparts forming a netting of the collagen in your cartilage. Now, further imagine that hundreds of microscopic bottle brushes, each with dozens of bristles, are nestling in the interstices of the netting. These are the *proteoglycans* that soak up and hold fluid in the cartilage, allowing it to flow in and out as the pressure on a joint decreases and increases.

3. J. F. Fries, "Assessing and Understanding Patient Risk," *Scan J Rheumatol* 92, suppl. (1992): 21–24.

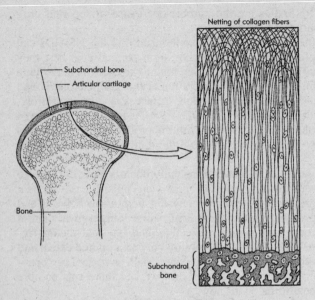

Figure 1. Cartilage

The fluid gives cartilage its resiliency, ability to absorb pressure, and surface slipperiness.

As previously stated, cartilage protects the ends of bones, letting them work smoothly together in a joint. Collagen forms the cartilage matrix that holds the proteoglycans in place. Proteoglycans ''drink in'' the cushioning and nourishing fluid. It's here, deep within the cartilage, that osteoarthritis begins. And it's here that the arthritis cure's key components set things right. Spearheaded by the two natural, nutritional supplements, glucosamine and chondroitin sulfates, the program described in this book rebuilds the internal structure of the cartilage so that it once again becomes strong and healthy.

The Arthritis Cure Revisited

Today, there is no question that this combination of supplements, as described in *The Arthritis Cure,* works. It intuitively makes sense that they would, since these substances are already found in strong, healthy joints. There is also a whole new body of research that proves their efficacy. This evidence, which includes double-blind studies that have been conducted in prestigious health centers around the world, is incontrovertible.

But most important, we've seen *The Arthritis Cure* work in numerous patients. Many of them had been told by their doctors that there was no hope of improvement and that they were doomed to a lifetime of pain, side effects from medications, possible surgery, and eventual disability. Not pleasant prospects, but the best that standard medicine had to offer.

The Maximizing Program

Glucosamine and chondroitin are an essential part of treating osteoarthritis. However, they alone cannot solve the whole problem. To achieve the full effect, they have to be used in conjunction with a correct biomechanical program to minimize further wear and tear on the joints, an appropriate eating plan to add the nutrients the joints need, and a simple regime of additional supplements to make glucosamine/chondroitin more effective. Thus, to ensure that glucosamine/chondroitin work to their maximum advantage, we developed a nine-point program that we presented in *The Arthritis Cure* and that we are now augmenting with the more recent findings. To truly maximize the effectiveness of the cure, we therefore urge you to follow these nine points.

1. Consult your physician in depth. In Chapter 3, we discuss how your doctor will reach a diagnosis, what sort of ques-

tions you can expect to be asked, and how to get the most out of this consultation.

2. Take glucosamine and chondroitin sulfates to repair damaged joints. In Chapter 9, we discuss other supplements that may enhance their effectiveness.

3. Understand and implement the principles of biomechanics to minimize ongoing stress to your joints. We discuss how to do this in Chapter 4.

4. Do the right sort of exercise regularly. We give you a detailed program that you can tailor to your personal needs in Chapter 5.

5. Eat a healthful, joint-preserving diet, making a special effort to include foods that contain nutrients that are of particular value to arthritis sufferers. We show you how to do this in Chapter 6 and even suggest a few recipes to prove that eating correctly can taste great.

6. Maintain your ideal body weight. This is, of course, a function of following a diet and exercise program that is appropriate for you, as provided in these pages.

7. Help overcome or avoid depression by staying active. Clearly, solving the main part of your arthritis problem— and knowing that you *can* solve it—goes a long way to resolve any depressive symptoms you may be feeling.

8. Use traditional medicines as necessary. There is a place for them, though many will find their use unnecessary by following the rest of the arthritis cure program. There are some promising new prescription treatments for both osteo- and rheumatoid arthritis that we'll discuss in Chapters 7, 8, and 9.

9. Maintain a positive attitude. Your arthritis can be helped. Optimistic and hopeful mental attitudes can make a real difference in the body due to the mind-body interaction.

Now let us examine some of these nine points in a little more detail, before moving on to your full program of maximizing the arthritis cure, to clarify their roles and emphasize their importance.

Consult Your Physician

At first glance, it should seem obvious that any treatment of a disease or condition that is as severe as arthritis ought to be discussed with your doctor. While the arthritis cure described in this book is perfectly safe for the vast majority of people the vast majority of the time, only your doctor knows whether it is fully compatible with your overall state of health. Only your doctor and you can decide what treatment is appropriate for you.

Glucosamine

Glucosamine, which has several important functions in the joints, is produced in small quantities in the body from glucose and amino acids. It can also be ingested in very small quantities through certain foods. This natural substance stimulates the production of and serves as raw material for the water-loving proteoglycans, and other special proteins called glycosaminoglycans (GAGs) that bind water in the cartilage matrix. Glucosamine also regulates cartilage metabolism, helping to keep cartilage build-up and break-down mechanisms balanced. This, in turn, helps prevent untimely or unnecessary tissue loss. Studies conducted all around the world have proved that glucosamine reduces pain and improves the joint function disrupted by osteoarthritis, all the while strengthening the body's natural repair mechanisms. (For more information on these studies see Appendix A.)

Glucosamine not only successfully quells pain and other symptoms of osteoarthritis, it does so more effectively than ibuprofen, the active ingredient in Advil, Motrin, Nuprin, and other popular arthritis remedies. In a double-blind study comparing glucosamine to ibuprofen in forty osteoarthritis patients, both medications began by relieving pain well. At first, it seemed as if ibuprofen was more effective than glucosamine, but after two weeks, ibuprofen's benefits seemed to wane. (This often happens with drugs as the body, and perhaps the mind, becomes habituated to them and experiences fewer benefits.) The glucosamine, however, continued strong. When the

eight-week study was concluded, the pain score for the glucosamine group was about a third of that in the ibuprofen
group.[4] Studies in other laboratories confirm that glucosamine
is at least as effective as ibuprofen, if not more so, and much
better tolerated.[5]

Chondroitin

By itself, glucosamine is a powerful tool against osteoarthritis.
But it's only half of the amazing team of natural substances
that offer a way to healthy joints.

Remember the proteoglycan molecules that embed themselves in the spaces in the collagen netting that gives structure
to the cartilage in joints? Imagine that you're looking into the
proteoglycans. You'll see "trees," with numerous branches
jutting out from the trunk. Growing out of each of the branches
are about a hundred smaller branches made of long chains of
chondroitin sulfates. It's these chondroitin chains in the proteoglycans that actually draw in the cushioning and nourishing
synovial fluid. Chondroitin sulfates also help prevent prema-
ture breakdown of cartilage in two ways: They stop the naturally occurring enzymes from going haywire and actually
"chewing" up cartilage; and they inhibit other enzymes from
shutting off the flow of nutrients to the cartilage.

Glucosamine Plus Chondroitin Sulfates, the One-Two Punch

As discussed more fully in The Arthritis Cure, a great deal of
experimental evidence and clinical experience has confirmed
that glucosamine and chondroitin sulfates are indeed the be-
ginnings of a powerful new arthritis treatment. Since the pub-

---

4. A. L. Vaz, "Double-blind Clinical Evaluation of the Relative Efficacy of
Ibuprofen and Glucosamine Sulphate in the Management of Osteoarthritis of
the Knee in Out-patients," Current Medical Research and Opinion 8, no. 3
(1982): 145–49.
5. See, for example, H. M. Fassbender et al., "Glucosamine Sulphate Compared to Ibuprofen in Osteoarthritis of the Knee," Osteoarthritis and Cartilage 2, no. 1 (1994): 61–69.

lication of that book, additional research has confirmed those findings. Together, these two natural nutritional supplements increase the production of proteoglycans, GAGs, and other key elements of healthy cartilage; enhance the manufacture of hyaluronate, which makes joint fluid viscous and able to lubricate joints; slow the enzymes that needlessly break down cartilage tissue or interfere with the flow of nutrients; help ''clean up'' cholesterol, fibrin, fats, and other deposits in joints and nearby blood vessels; reduce pain; and improve mobility. At last, osteoarthritis victims can look forward to less pain, stronger joints, *and* the prospect of complete recovery.

There are many possible reasons you may feel skeptical. One reason is that there have been many ultimately disappointing claims about new arthritis treatments. None of these, however, was able to stand up to the most rigorous of scientific scrutiny in double-blind, controlled human studies. But the individual treatments recommended in *The Arthritis Cure* have withstood such rigorous testing. This treatment is not just the latest fad. We have challenged the medical community with a new program, and it is quickly becoming the standard for treating arthritis and avoiding the potentially dangerous, and sometimes even lethal, side effects of current treatments.

You may resist accepting the precepts laid out in *The Arthritis Cure* because adopting new ideas is challenging; it's easier to cling to what we've been taught and always believed to be true. But remember, most things we now consider routine in medicine were at one time considered odd, even threatening. Even the idea of washing hands before surgery was once considered shocking and insulting to doctors!

Finally, you may be one of a group of people, and that includes some doctors, who simply don't trust studies that come from other countries, incorrectly believing that only American studies conducted by American scientists are valid. The truth, of course, is that many scientific and medical advances emanate from overseas. If you need proof of this, remember that penicillin was discovered by a Scottish scientist, and we have safe milk thanks to a French chemist.

A Note for the Skeptic

Previously, the only legitimate criticism of the program was that there had not yet been double-blind studies utilizing *both* glucosamine and chondroitin sulfates. This has now changed, as two new U.S. studies using the supplements have been completed. Of course, individually, each of these supplements has been proved to be effective against osteoarthritis in carefully conducted research studies. Clinically, we have found a much more effective response in patients taking both supplements (in a 5:4 ratio) than in the same patients taking one or the other supplement alone.

Biomechanics

Part of exercise is increasing your body's ability to perform the tasks you want it to. But another part, which we call biomechanics, is teaching your body to perform those tasks efficiently, with the minimum wear and tear.

We all know that if you incorrectly lift a heavy object, you are likely to put your back out. And we are all fully aware that if you get hit hard by a large and heavy object, you will likely suffer some damage. If that damage happens to be to cartilage, then we know that osteoarthritis may start at the damaged point. But we are less aware—and often quite ignorant—that very small traumas, constantly repeated, can add up to equally problematic damage and may also lead to osteoarthritis. Thus, jolting up and down stairs, and subjecting knee cartilage to constant banging as we land on stair after stair, year after year, may cause just as much damage as being subjected to a painful kick during a football game. And the resultant arthritis of the knee may become even more painful and severe.

Of course, you cannot eliminate *all* everyday joint trauma. And there is no need to give up your favorite sports. However, you can minimize trauma by learning how to disperse the shocks your body receives over the broadest area possible. When you walk down a flight of stairs, your joints actually carry three to five times your body weight. When you squat, they may be carrying ten to twenty times your weight. And if you squat down, then lift a heavy object . . . well, you get the idea. Clearly, if these pressures are not dispersed, but instead are concentrated on only a small cross section of your joints, they are likely to cause small injuries. Such injuries, repeated incessantly, almost inevitably lead to osteoarthritis.

Biomechanics, then, is the art of moving, standing, sitting, and even lying down correctly. It is not automatic, but once learned, it becomes second nature. And improving your body's biomechanics is an important part of maximizing the arthritis cure.

Exercise

The benefits of exercise are not limited to the joints. Exercise improves overall physical health and capability, contributes to self-esteem and emotional wellness, reduces stress while promoting relaxation, enhances sleep, builds muscle while "melting" body fat, improves sexual function and satisfaction, and helps us preserve our ability to live independently well into old age. Not exercising, on the other hand, increases the risk of developing heart disease, elevated blood pressure, diabetes, and obesity. (After smoking, a sedentary lifestyle is felt to be the second leading, underlying cause of disease and death in the United States.)

Certain types of exercise are also good for bones, making them thicker and stronger. *Weight-bearing exercise* does this by forcing your bones to work against gravity. As you walk, jog, or run, for example, your feet, legs, and hips carry the weight of your body. The bones in the lower part of the body respond by growing stronger and thicker. *Strength training* not only builds muscle but also strengthens bones. Lifting weights puts a burden on the muscles and bones involved in moving and suppporting that weight, thus increasing their bulk and strength.

A Healthful Diet, a Healthful Weight

One of the essential therapies for osteoarthritis, and indeed for all arthritic conditions, is regular, healthful eating. Selecting a variety of nutritionally sound foods with the right complement of vitamins, minerals, and antioxidants, and then cooking them properly, helps you maintain long-term health. The right choices can also help prevent lethargy, feelings of melancholy, and depression.

One of the best medicines for osteoarthritis is weight loss, if you are overweight. This is especially true if your pain is in the hips, knees, spine, or other weight-bearing joints. Even if the osteoarthritis is in a non-weight-bearing joint, such as the elbow, losing weight may still be beneficial, for it improves overall health and may lower the levels of some of the chemicals in the blood that have been implicated in osteoarthritis.

Unfortunately, losing weight is easier said than done, so many people turn to quick, "magic" weight-loss programs. As a result, weight loss is a multibillion-dollar industry, with diet books, diet centers, diet drugs, special foods, and slimming apparatuses of all sorts touted constantly. Most of these approaches to dieting work temporarily, but then tend to boomerang on the dieter. As millions of disgusted dieters have found, it's much easier to lose weight than to keep it off. Within a few months, and often a lot sooner, most regain all the weight they lost—and often more. Besides the indignity of weighing more than ever, many dieters find that they now have new health problems caused by their diet.

As we discuss in Chapter 6, there are better ways of dieting than following fads. Good solid eating is what it's all about, and that includes eating excellent, tasty meals. No one but a fanatic can stick for long to an all-cabbage diet, or any diet that leaves you permanently hungry. We believe in healthful eating: the consumption of well-balanced, delicious meals full of important nutrients in reasonably moderate portions.

In Summary

There is a lot of new and useful material in this book. For example, Chapter 9 describes a great deal of new information about several nutrients, some of them just now emerging, that promise to be of great help in alleviating arthritis symptoms. For example, a European breakthrough, S-Adenosyl methionine (nicknamed SAMe, "Sammy" to its friends), seems to have major antiarthritis benefits; and an exciting supplement called hydrolyzed collagen is expected to have beneficial effects on damaged cartilage. You will also learn of several other promising agents, new surgical techniques, specifics on how to improve your biomechanics, and more. Above all, however, you will learn how to implement the program we just recapped for you in this chapter to greatest possible effect. All told, *Maximizing the Arthritis Cure* does just that. As a result, you will be able to deal with your arthritis problems to an extent never before possible.

Let's begin with a look at ways to work effectively with your doctor in diagnosing and treating your arthritis. Once you know how to do that, you are well on the way to knowing how to maximize the cure, while tailoring it to your personal lifestyle.

3

Working with Your Physician

Glucosamine and chondroitin sulfates, the two supplements that spearhead the arthritis cure, have received a great deal of attention. Deservedly so, since they offer for the first time ever an opportunity actually to repair damaged cartilage and begin to cure osteoarthritis. But maximizing the cure is a little more complex than just taking two pills and not bothering to call your doctor in the morning. Glucosamine and chondroitin sulfates may quickly relieve your symptoms, but before deciding on any course of treatment you should first see a physician to verify that you do indeed have osteoarthritis. Because osteoarthritis is a complicated problem affecting us on both physical and emotional levels, it requires careful diagnosis and treatment. And it's important for doctor and patient to work carefully together, whether the case is minor or advanced.

The process begins with the clinical diagnosis. There is no single test, like a blood or urine test, that can pinpoint whether you have osteoarthritis. In order to make such a diagnosis, the physician must conduct a thorough examination that consists of taking a detailed medical history, performing a complete physical examination, and ordering X rays or other imaging studies that let your doctor ''see'' the state of your disease.

Step 1: The Discussion

Modern technology has produced an astonishing number of impressive diagnostic tools. With computerized axial tomography (CAT) scans and magnetic resonance imaging (MRI), we can ''see'' right into the human body. Angiography allows us to follow special dyes as they flow through tiny arteries in the heart. And with new experimental laboratory techniques, we can find small clusters of cancerous cells hidden among millions of healthy cells.

Despite these high-tech tools, there's nothing quite as useful as a long conversation between doctor and patient. The most important component of this conversation, especially for diagnosing osteoarthritis, is the medical history taken by the doctor. During this talk, the careful doctor asks many open-ended questions designed to get you talking. Questions that require yes or no answers will not do. Here are some of the things he or she will want to know. You may want to think about them before your visit so that your responses are accurate and complete. You may even want to copy these pages and write down your answers. That will save you both time. The clearer and more concise your answers, the better able your doctor will be to make an accurate diagnosis.

Taking Your Medical History

In order to determine that you have osteoarthritis, as distinct from some other condition or illness that may have the same symptoms, your doctor will want to know a lot about the type of pain, stiffness, swelling, and other symptoms you are experiencing. The following are the main areas about which you will probably be questioned.

PAIN   Although pain is the hallmark of osteoarthritis, it can be caused by a bewildering variety of other diseases, conditions, and injuries. It is therefore vital that the doctor ask numerous questions to make sure that your pain is being caused by osteoarthritis, not another problem. The location of the pain, its severity, character, timing, and other qualities help your doctor to establish the proper diagnosis and guide you toward the right treatment. The questions are likely to include:

- *Where does it hurt? In a specific part of the joint, or the whole area?* Osteoarthritis pain is often localized to the joint that hurts, but there are some classic patterns of radiating pain—such as from neck to shoulder, hip to knee, back to buttocks—so the place that hurts may not be the place that is causing the pain, and the cause of the pain may not be osteoarthritis.

- *How does it hurt? Is your pain sharp, burning, aching, stabbing, or throbbing?* In the initial stages of osteoarthritis, people often feel a throbbing pain, like a toothache. Later in the course of the disease, sharp or stabbing pains can coexist with the throbbing. A burning type pain is uncommon in osteoarthritis.

- *When do you hurt? All the time, after certain activities, after resting?* With osteoarthritis, rest usually provides short-term relief of pain.

- *Is it worse in the morning, afternoon, evening, or night?* Pain from osteoarthritis so severe that it wakes a person is often due to an advanced stage of the disease. Such pain may also be caused by an unusual amount of inflammation, which raises the suspicion that there is more than osteoarthritis involved.

- *Do different kinds of exercise make it feel worse? Better?* If the pain is worse after exercise, it may be due to joint alignment problems. Alternatively, if the pain tends to lessen after exercise, this suggests a need to improve muscle tone.

- *How long have you had the pain?* Osteo and other forms of arthritis are diagnosed after the pain has been present in a joint for a minimum of two consecutive weeks.

- *Did you suffer an injury or illness shortly before the pain began, or did it just happen spontaneously?* Muscle pulls, bone bruises, and ligament and other injuries can mimic the pain of osteoarthritis.

- *Did you gain or lose weight in the year or so before the pain began?* Weight gain often worsens symptoms of most forms of arthritis. However, weight gain can also precipitate a sudden, severe attack of gout due to a build-up of uric acid crystals in a joint. Your doctor has to differentiate between these two conditions. Weight loss should improve symptoms. However, significant weight loss, especially in an older individual who did not do anything to lose the weight, may indicate more severe problems that should immediately be brought to the attention of your doctor.
- *Was the pain initially mild, becoming worse over time, or was it severe right from the start?* Osteoarthritis is rarely severe from the start. Therefore, an early onset of severe pain suggests that this pain may stem from other causes.
- *If the pain began mildly and increased, has the increase been slow and steady, or did it suddenly become worse?* Except for osteoarthritis due to an acute injury, slow and steady is the general developmental pattern. A different progression of pain suggests that there may be problems other than osteoarthritis involved.

STIFFNESS   Joint stiffness, which can be physically and emotionally troubling, is often an indication of arthritis. No other conditions cause exactly the same type of joint stiffness as osteoarthritis. Therefore, your doctor may probe to determine as closely as possible exactly what your particular feeling of stiffness involves.

- *Does the affected joint feel stiff?* Think about this question for a moment. People often confuse stiffness with voluntary restriction of movement due to pain, which is a different symptom.
- *If so, is it stiff at a particular time? In the morning, after exercise or certain movements, after resting, or after sitting for long periods?* This is an important diagnostic question

because rheumatoid arthritis generally causes you to experience morning stiffness, which sometimes lasts for half an hour or more. Joint stiffness from osteoarthritis can occur whenever you stop moving the joint for a while, though the stiffness disappears in seconds or minutes after movement is recommenced.

- *Is the stiffness always the same, or are there times when your joints feel stiffer?* How you answer this question can provide useful diagnostic clues. For example, advanced cases of osteoarthritis can result in permanent limitations in movement, whereas even in fairly severe rheumatoid arthritis, joint stiffness tends to be more variable than in osteoarthritis.

SWELLING   In approximately 85 to 90 percent of osteoarthritis cases, inflammation is not a problem. Still, it's important to ask about it because the presence of swelling can indicate the degree of joint damage or suggest that there's another problem either masquerading as osteoarthritis or in addition to it. Joint infections can lead to swelling. So can gout (uric acid crystals), pseudogout (calcium crystals), and bursitis. A single joint that becomes swollen suddenly must have fluid drawn for analysis. Seeing a physician and getting some of the excess fluid withdrawn and analyzed can very accurately pinpoint the diagnosis of either of these crystalline deposit diseases.

- *Is the swollen joint painful and stiff?* A swollen joint may be stiff or painful because of the excess fluid in it, which can impede movement.
- *Did the pain, stiffness, and swelling begin at the same time?* Such a concurrence of symptoms is often found in an acute injury or in crystalline joint disease.
- *Does alcohol, or short-term weight gain, sometimes trigger the swelling?* These symptoms are factors in gout more often than in osteoarthritis.
- *Is there more swelling in the morning, afternoon, evening, or night?* Swelling from osteoarthritis is often greatest after you have been using the joint all day, since the prolonged

rubbing of the bones together causes a temporary inflammation.

SEVERITY The degree of which you are suffering is important. Not only does it suggest the extent of joint damage, it also hints at how much treatment you may need, and how soon. Of course, joint pain is rarely if ever constant, so you need to think of the average lows and highs for the pain. To get an overall sense of your situation, your doctor might ask something like, "How would you rate your pain on a scale of zero to ten, with zero being no pain and ten being the worse pain you have ever felt?" Thereafter, you could expect the following types of questions:

- *Are you having difficulty working?* If you are, your doctor may recommend switching to a less arduous job, at least until your condition improves. This applies especially to jobs that involve light impact on joints such as certain construction jobs, jackhammer operations, or heavy-lifting factory work.
- *Is the pain, stiffness, and/or swelling preventing you from exercising, participating in sports, or performing leisure activities?* If it is, you should not stop exercising, but you may wish to modify your exercise program. There is no need or benefit from doing something you find really painful.
- *Is pain interfering with your self-care and other everyday activities?* If so, you clearly have a very serious problem that needs prompt and thorough treatment.
- *Do you have difficulty walking or standing?* If so, you may need assisting devices such as a walking stick or a full walker.

CAUSATION Knowing, for example, that you suffered an injury before the pain began can be a valuable clue that you are suffering from secondary osteoarthritis, whereas if no injury occurred, you are more likely to have primary osteoarthritis. Information about your family medical history can also be very helpful, as certain types of arthritis run in families. And it is important to know which types because they may have an impact on your condition, masking or aggravating some symptoms. Therefore, your doctors may ask:

- *Can you remember anything that happened—injury, illness, surgery, significant weight gain or loss—shortly before your pain began or got worse?* Interestingly, inflammatory forms of arthritis such as rheumatoid arthritis and lupus often become symptomatic after some emotionally traumatic or stressful event.
- *Does anyone else in your family—grandparents, parents, uncles, aunts, or siblings—have the same or similar pain?* If so, there is a possibility of an inherited condition. Such knowledge may lead to a quicker diagnosis of your condition.
- *Does anyone in your family have arthritis?* Some kinds of arthritis have a clear hereditary component. Osteoarthritis of the hands, rheumatoid arthritis, lupus, gout, and other forms seem to run in families.
- *Are you taking any medicines, whether prescribed for you, purchased over the counter, or given to you by a friend? This includes any herbal or vitamin/mineral supplements.* Medication use may mask certain diagnostic clues. It is very important that doctors know down to the pill what medications and/or vitamins you are taking.
- *Were you taking any medicines before or just when the problem began?* Sometimes, adverse reactions to medications can lead to joint pain.

GENERAL HEALTH   Rheumatoid arthritis and other forms of the disease can cause joint symptoms that at first glance seem similar to those of osteoarthritis. Or the situation may be confused because you may have both osteo- and rheumatoid arthritis. There also are diseases that can coexist with osteoarthritis, and they often have their own unique symptoms. The presence of one or more of these symptoms can help to indicate what conditions other than osteoarthritis may be present. That's why your physician will ask questions about your general health and mood.

- *Have you been feeling less energetic lately?* This symptom is more often associated with the inflammatory forms of arthritis, such as rheumatoid arthritis, than with osteoarthritis.
- *Are you experiencing fevers, or have you been sweating more than usual, especially at night?* Again, this is more common with RA than osteoarthritis.
- *Have you been having difficulty sleeping?* If so, this may account for your feeling more pain, since poor sleep patterns tend to lower your pain threshold.
- *Have you changed your diet recently?* Some diets, for example, those high in red meats, can worsen inflammatory types of arthritis. A vegetarian diet has been shown to help some patients with rheumatoid arthritis.
- *Have you had any recent changes in your bowel habits?* Chronic diarrhea may be due to celiac disease (an intestinal intolerance to gluten, a protein found in wheat, rye, barley, and oats). The best treatment is dietary avoidance of gluten-containing products.
- *Are you feeling weak (i.e., are you having difficulty lifting heavy objects or exerting yourself physically)?* Obviously, weakness can be caused by any number of diseases, but once your doctor has pinpointed your problem as arthritis, this symptom of weakness points to one of these inflammatory types of arthritis where it is more common than in osteoarthritis.
- *Have you had pink eye, dry eyes, or other eye problems?* These symptoms can occur in some types of arthritis, such as Reiter's syndrome and Sjögren's syndrome.
- *Have you had any sores or dryness in your mouth?* Answering yes to this or the preceding questions may suggest the possibility of rheumatoid arthritis, Reiter's syndrome, psoriatic arthritis, or other forms of arthritis. Your doctor will then have to tease apart your various symptoms in order to determine whether you are also suffering from osteoarthritis.

OTHER CONDITIONS As part of determining your general health, it is of course vital that your physician know what other diseases or conditions you have or might have. These diseases may be causing your pain, stiffness, and/or swelling, and they may interfere with your treatment. That is why the doctor will ask questions such as:

- *Do you have, or have you had, any other diseases? Heart disease, diabetes, high blood pressure, or kidney problems?* Certain constellations of conditions can point to a particular form of arthritis.
- *Have these been diagnosed and treated by another physician?* Sometimes various conditions have not been pieced together and understood to be emanating from the same basic disorder.
- *Are you taking any medicines, undergoing therapy, eating a special diet, doing special exercises, or otherwise being treated for these diseases?* If so, your doctor needs to know the details in order to be sure that your osteoarthritis program is compatible with your other treatment.
- *Have you had any surgeries? If so, on what part of the body, when, and why?* Previous surgery can have a profound effect on the development of osteoarthritis since any trauma to a joint, including its surgical repair, can be the precursor of osteoarthritis.

The Answers Are in the Questions

It is vital that the doctor ask you many questions, then carefully consider your answers, since a variety of problems can be causing or contributing to your pain. A doctor who makes a quick diagnosis of osteoarthritis when you say your back hurts, for example, may be missing a number of potential problems, from a strained muscle, to kidney disease, to cancer.

We cannot overstate the importance of the doctor-patient conversation. Throughout the ages, wise physicians have said over and over again that patients will guide their doctors to their problems—if only the doctors will ask the right questions and listen carefully to their patients' answers.

Again, you can help your doctor by reviewing the questions above before going in for an examination. Think about your symptoms, when they began, when they wax and wane, what seems to make them worse. Try to remember what illnesses, injuries, or surgeries you have had. Look through copies of any medical records you have to refresh your memory. If you're going to be seen by a new doctor, arrange to have your medical records sent over from your previous physician before the first examination. Otherwise, your diagnosis and the beginning of treatment may have to wait several days or weeks until your medical records have arrived and been studied. Usually you have to sign a "release of medical record form" before your records can be sent from one facility to another, so plan ahead.

Some physicians will send you a lengthy questionnaire to fill out before the first examination. You will find its instructions similar to the ones we are listing, so use the doctor's questionnaire to remain consistent with his or her other patients, but add any additional information we have listed as important. Although filling out a questionnaire may seem to be a tedious chore, we urge you to do it completely, using additional sheets of paper if necessary to jot down as much of your personal and family medical history as you can remember. Items you may think are not important or are unrelated are often quite valuable to the doctor. More content—although perhaps not more words—is definitely better.

Questions to Ask Your Doctor(s)

Just as it is essential that your doctor ask you questions, it is important that you question your doctor. In order to cooperate fully in whatever program of healing your doctor prescribes, you must be fully informed. Your doctor should be an excellent source of information, so ask about your symptoms as well as the therapies, medicines, or surgeries he or she is suggesting. No question is too "silly" or "unimportant" to ask. You have the right to know, and your doctor has the obligation to inform you. So don't hesitate. After all, talking to patients is part of the job that physicians are paid to do. Moreover, many doctors understand that the more their patients know, the more comfortable and cooperative they will be. Indeed, although few people realize it, in our experience, most doctors much prefer to treat people who are educated about their illness and motivated toward getting healthy—even if it means that the physician has to spend a little more time answering questions.

Getting Organized

The arthritis cure begins as soon as you make an appointment with your doctor. Before your appointment, gather the information the doctor will need and think about questions you want answered. Here are some useful steps:

- Contact any other doctors, clinics, chiropractors, or other health professionals of whom you've been a patient, to have your medical records forwarded to your current physician. (Your doctor will undoubtedly do this after you've seen him or her, but it's best to have those records available when you first visit your doctor, not later. Yes, this may inundate your physician with information, but that's better than not having enough, or not having it when it's most important.)
- Prepare notes on when your pain, stiffness, or other problems strike, what you're doing at the time these symptoms occur, and how intense the problem is. By referring to the previous section of this chapter, you can check what your doctor will want to know, making it quite easy for you to list your answers.
- Make a list of all medications (prescription and over-the-counter), supplements, or herbs you are taking. (Most pharmacies keep patient records on computer. Ask your pharmacist to print out a complete list of all the medicines you have taken.) Also list the amount of alcohol you consume and whether you smoke.
- Make a list of all treatments, even home remedies, you've undergone.

Here are some of the many questions you should ask. The point is not to give your doctor(s) the third degree. Rather, it is to learn as much as you can about your body and to assure yourself that you are getting the best possible treatment. It is quite possible, of course, that your doctor will prefer to answer your questions during a follow-up visit, by which time he or she will have your test results and will know more about your condition.

GENERAL QUESTIONS

- What made you conclude that I have osteoarthritis?
- Can my symptoms have been caused by other diseases or conditions?
- If I do have osteoarthritis, is it primary or secondary (i.e., the result of some other condition)?
- If it is secondary osteoarthritis, what other types of treatments could help eliminate the cause of the problem?
- Is there any joint deformity? If so, please tell me where and to what degree.
- Are there any bony spurs? If so, where?
- Are there any Heberden's nodes? If so, where?
- Which treatment do you recommend? Why?

IF YOUR DOCTOR SUGGESTS DRUG TREATMENT

- Exactly which medicine(s) do you recommend?
- How often should it be taken?
- When should it be taken?
- Should I eat before taking the medicine?
- Are there any foods or beverages I should restrict or eliminate altogether while taking this drug?
- Are there any activities I should modify or restrict while taking this medicine?
- What are the major possible side effects, and what should I do if they occur?
- Will this medicine interfere with any other treatment I am currently receiving?

- What exactly does this medicine do? Relieve pain? Reduce inflammation?
- How long before I can expect this medicine to take effect?
- If it does not work, will you then suggest other medicines? Which ones?
- Will this medicine actually cure my osteoarthritis, or will it only mask my pain?
- If it's intended only to mask the pain, do I really need it? Will physical therapy, exercise, or a change in lifestyle reduce the pain instead?

IF YOUR DOCTOR SUGGESTS PHYSICAL THERAPY

- Exactly what kind of therapy are you recommending (heat, massage, hydrotherapy, special exercises, etc.)?
- Why this therapy? What are we hoping will be accomplished?
- Exactly what will be done to me?
- Who will perform this therapy?
- How long will it last?
- How long before I should expect to feel better?
- How will we know if it's working?
- Will this help me long term, or is this just a short-term comfort therapy?

IF YOUR DOCTOR SUGGESTS SURGERY

- What surgery are you recommending?
- Please describe what happens during this surgery.
- What outcome are you hoping for? In other words, exactly how will I be better off as a result of this surgery?
- What is the normal range of outcomes from this type of surgery?
- Please describe all the side effects of this surgery, from the most common to the least. What percent of your patients suffer from these side effects?
- How long will I be in the hospital following surgery?
- Will I be in pain after the surgery? To what extent, for how

long, and what can be done to relieve that pain, if necessary?

- Will I be laid up or unable to care for myself following the surgery? Should I arrange to have someone help me when I return home?
- Will the surgery affect my ability to work? To what extent, and for how long? Can anything be done to help me get back to work sooner, if that's necessary?
- In what hospital will the surgery be performed?
- Is that hospital noted for good surgical results? Are there any statistics or ratings to show that?
- Do you have any books or pamphlets describing this surgery?
- Do you have any patients who have undergone the treatment you recommend who would be willing to talk with me?
- Can this surgery significantly affect or cure my osteoarthritis?
- Could the surgery make my condition worse than it is now?

OTHER IMPORTANT QUESTIONS TO ASK REGARDING YOUR TREATMENT

- Who will be in overall charge of my treatment, you or another doctor?
- If other doctors are involved, how will you communicate and work with each other?
- What will my treatment cost? Will your office staff help me fill out my insurance papers?
- Is another treatment other than the one you recommend suitable for me? Why or why not?
- What will happen if I do nothing but ask you to keep an eye on the problem for a while?
- What alternative therapies are available? Please describe them to me.

ASK YOUR DOCTOR ABOUT THE ARTHRITIS CURE

- Are you aware of glucosamine and chondroitin sulfates?
- How about the other important principles in this book—

biomechanics, exercise, diet, and other promising supplements?
- What if I were to take chondroitin and glucosamine and the other recommended supplements instead of the therapy you suggest?
- What if I were to take them in addition to the therapy you suggest?

Step 2: The Physical Examination

Even if the discussion suggests that you have osteoarthritis, the careful doctor will still perform a complete physical examination from head to toe. He or she will look at your general appearance, checking for unusual marks, bruises, discoloration, or other potential problems; listen to your heart and lungs; peer into your eyes, ears, and mouth; probe your belly; measure your blood pressure and weight; check your grip strength; and otherwise evaluate your general health.

You may wonder why the doctor doesn't simply focus on the part of your body that's hurting. After all, osteoarthritis does not affect the heart or lungs, nor does it affect your hearing or vision. The examination must be thorough because there are many reasons for pain. Pain is a complicated and potentially misleading symptom. Sometimes the key piece of evidence that establishes a diagnosis can be found in some internal organ, not in the joint that hurts. For example, osteoarthritis of the spine can cause back pain. But a very similar pain can result from kidney stones, a herniated disk, or menstrual problems. Arthritis may be producing the pain in your knee, or it might be caused by tendinitis or bursitis. The signs and symptoms of many diseases overlap, making them difficult to sort out without a careful conversation and examination.

To complicate matters even more, the pain we feel does not always ''come from'' where we think it does. Pain is often ''referred'' from one part of the body to another. For example, problems with the back are often felt as pains in the hips. Hip disease can be felt in the groin and sometimes even in the knees.

Following the routine, general examination, the doctor will inspect your joints with his or her eyes and hands, checking to see how mobile they are, whether or not they are stable, and how much (if any) pain you feel on active and passive movement. Depending on what joints are affected, the doctor may ask you to stand up, walk around, sit down, lift your arms, bend over, reach out, and so on. He or she may test your strength in the area under question by asking you to do something like raise your leg while he or she pushes down on it in order to establish whether your muscles, not just sore joints, have problems. Your doctor may also use a tape measure to see if the muscles or joints in one limb are larger than those in the other.

The complexity of the history and physical findings related to pain is the reason it is necessary to see a doctor who is trained to sort out the subtle differences from condition to condition. Only in that way can you be sure all your pain stems from osteoarthritis and can therefore be treated by the arthritis cure.

Step 3: X Rays

Your doctor will most likely have made a preliminary diagnosis of osteoarthritis based on your conversation and physical examination. The next step is to order X rays of the afflicted joint(s), looking for the characteristic physical degeneration of the bone ends to confirm the diagnosis (see Figure 2).

But X rays are just one part of the process and do not necessarily provide conclusive evidence. The physical damage they show is not always directly related to the degree of pain; stiffness and disability are not always related to the amount of physical damage. Some people in great distress show little or no evidence of osteoarthritis on X rays, while others with significantly damaged joints suffer relatively little stress.

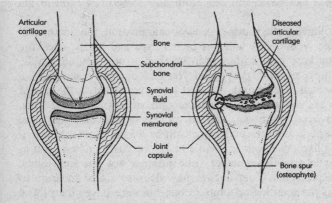

Figure 2. Healthy and Unhealthy Joints

If your doctor skimps on either the conversation or the physical examination and attempts to diagnose or rule out osteoarthritis on the basis of X rays alone, find yourself another doctor. Missing a treatable cause of your joint pain may forever adversely alter your life. You cannot afford to treat this matter casually.

Step 4: Other Tests

Thorough discussion, physical examination, and X rays are usually enough to make a diagnosis of osteoarthritis. Occasionally, however, more tests such as blood or urine analyses are called for—not to show that you have osteoarthritis but to rule out other conditions that may be causing your symptoms. You may have some symptoms of osteoarthritis along with others that suggest another problem. Careful doctors keep investigating until they are sure of the circumstances.

Assembling Your Team of Experts

If a diagnosis of osteoarthritis has been made, you're ready to begin treatment. Naturally, we recommend the nine-point program spearheaded by glucosamine and chondroitin sulfates and the enhancement program presented in this book. However, whether you use this or any other program, you are well-advised to continue working with your physician, so that he or she can monitor your progress and handle other things that may crop up.

Some people require more than monitoring; they need physical therapy or prescription medications for a time. And a small number require surgery to ''clean up'' damaged joints. Had you known about glucosamine and chondroitin when you felt your first symptoms, a lot of the care you may now need would probably not now be necessary. But you had no way of knowing. Consequently, you may have to deal with some major health issues in the future, and you may need a variety of experts to help you deal with them.

One of the great advantages of this book is that it can take the place of quite a bit of the health support you would need without it. Thus, the information a sound dietician normally provides is covered in Chapter 6; the know-how you need for optimum biochemical balance is provided in Chapter 4; and the advice you need to develop an appropriate exercise program is offered in Chapter 5. *Maximizing the Arthritis Cure* provides you with very complete information and as much health support as possible.

Obviously, however, no book can give you the diagnostic help, or the hands-on support that you can get from accredited experts. Thus, if your condition is severe, you still want to assemble your own health care team. With this book, you can better decide the kind of expert help you do need. And, best of all, you are equipped to evaluate their techniques and knowledge, and thus their ability to help you.

The experts to consider assembling for your team are:

- *Your physician,* who is most likely an internist, family practitioner, or geriatric specialist. It is very important that you maintain your relationship with this doctor and that you consult with and inform him or her about your treatment, even if it is being handled primarily by another specialist. Other physicians will come and go, but this is your primary doctor, the one who will help you care for your overall health. Let this doctor be your quarterback and coordinate your treatment, keeping track of what the others are doing, explaining everything to you, and looking out for your interests. If you move to another city, make it a priority to find a new primary doctor and have your complete medical records and history transferred promptly.
- *A registered dietitian,* who may help you lose weight, if necessary, and devise a healthful, joint-preserving diet. The precepts we lay down in Chapter 6 follow much the same diet as the one a dietitian could recommend. Therefore, you may feel that adding this person to your team is not essential.
- *A physical therapist,* who will teach you exercises to strengthen the muscles surrounding your afflicted joints. Here, too, the exercise program in this book should prove to be very similar to the one your physical therapist will recommend. Therefore, you will probably have little need for a physical therapist unless your condition is so severe that you need physical help to implement the exercises.

  Your therapist may also study the way you use your body, looking for ways that you might inadvertently be harming yourself by putting unnecessary pressure on your joints (i.e., give you a biomechanical analysis of what you are doing wrong). Once you have their diagnosis, you may find that our biomechanics discussion in Chapter 4 provides a full description of how to make any corrections you need.
- *An occupational therapist,* who can provide various devices—ranging from splints, to walkers, to special bottle openers—to help you function optimally at home and work.

- *An orthopedic surgeon,* who performs arthroscopic and other types of joint surgeries, including joint realignment and joint replacement. As we have emphasized, surgery should be the treatment of last resort and for only the most serious cases. Today, as noted, we know enough about glucosamine and chondroitin sulfates to help people developing the severity of osteoarthritis that requires surgery.

- *Practitioners of manipulative medicine* (osteopathic physicians, Rolfers, myotherapists, some but not all chiropractors, and physical therapists) can also help improve your biomechanics. However, once you have had a biomechanical analysis, "extra" professionals may not be necessary for you.

- *A psychiatrist or psychologist* to diagnose and treat any associated psychological conditions, such as the depression that is commonly associated with chronic pain and other life restrictions caused by this disease.

- *Alternative medicine specialists* (acupuncturists, herbalists, and even healing touch practitioners) could be part of your team if you feel you may gain a real benefit from them. Sometimes, these specialists can help you with specific aspects of osteoarthritis. For example, acupuncture can inhibit pain and may be useful while you wait for the glucosamine/chondroitin sulfates to become effective; herbs of various sorts may help with depression; and healing touch practitioners may provide the motivation to get started on the arthritis cure.

It is unlikely, of course, that you will need all of these professionals to deal with your problem. Indeed, many people have found glucosamine/chondroitin sulfates complemented with the other approaches explained in this book can halt or reverse their osteoarthritis. Nevertheless, it's good to be aware of the array of other health professionals whose expertise may help with the treatment of osteoarthritis. And any experts you do use will be especially valuable since you will know enough to use them effectively.

A Final Word

Whether you work with your family physician or a team of experts, always remember that *you* are the captain of the team. Your doctor and other health care experts have a great deal of information and expertise, but it's your body; you should make the decisions regarding its proper care. If someone is urging you to do something you have already decided against, stand firm. You are the boss. Your caregivers are highly trained and highly paid experts, but they are consultants who work for you.

Having been given a diagnosis of osteoarthritis by a physician, you will want to learn how to get the most out of the arthritis cure to solve your problems. In the next chapter, we discuss the second part of our nine-part program, how to use biomechanics to avoid further osteoarthritis damage and thus take a further step toward your ultimate cure, which is what this book is about.

4

Biomechanics, Stretching, and Balance

The single greatest cause of osteoarthritis is damage to joints. However, while most people think of damage as being the result of an accident or some direct trauma to their joints, the fact is that most damage is the result of a series of absurdly simple mistakes—standing, walking, bending, lifting, twisting, sitting, or lying incorrectly! If they are not done correctly, these normal movements, which we do over and over again, every day, year after year, can lead to joint problems.

The technical terms used by osteopathic physicians to describe the wear and tear on joints are *absolute overuse* and *relative overuse*. Absolute overuse occurs when specific activities are done incorrectly, or excessively, resulting in immediate damage. That is what happens when you lift a sofa and throw your back out. With reasonable care, you can avoid most cases of absolute overuse, although, of course, accidents do happen. Relative overuse is more difficult to guard against because it occurs when the forces applied by everyday activities are not evenly distributed throughout the body, resulting in subtle damage that becomes apparent only over time.

Consider, for instance, that you are carrying a heavy weight on your shoulder. It impacts not only your shoulder muscles and collarbone but also your spine, hips, thighs, knees, ankles, and feet. In this way, your body is analogous to a house with a heavy roof. Although the roof rests directly on several bearing walls, its weight is obviously transmitted through those walls right down into the foundation. If the bearing walls are not right above the foundation, or if the roof is not squarely on the bearing walls, the house will probably collapse. Similarly, the more evenly you stand when you carry that weight on your shoulder, the more dispersed the force of the weight becomes and the less pressure it places on any individual joint. Here is an everyday example. When you walk, your weight alternates from one leg to the other. If you are not correctly aligned straight up and down but instead have one hip jutting outward, then your body's weight is transmitted not through your whole leg but only through that part of it that is in the hip's direct path of force—probably your knee, and probably not right in the center of the knee where weight can be evenly distributed. If that force is excessive, it can quickly damage the knee. But more often this little wear and tear has a cumulative effect, leading eventually to osteoarthritis.

We should be clear that we are not talking here about *extra* weight, although that can be a factor, but about the force of the weight of your own body. That weight, bearing down on just part of a single joint (say, the outside of your knee) may well be doing your body lasting harm without your even noticing it—until one day you stand up and say, "Ouch!"

Biomechanics is the study of how the body deals with the relative overuse that is caused by force exerted both by the body's own weight and momentum, and by outside impact. If that force is channeled through a narrow pathway of joints or parts of joints, it is likely to cause damage, ultimately leading to osteoarthritis. However, if the force is dispersed through the largest possible number and expanse of bones, joints, and muscles, the damage is minimized. Thus, correct biomechanics is the art of positioning your body in such a way that all or at least most of the time it absorbs force or motion over as broad an area as possible. If your body is positioned in a biomechanically correct way, there is much less risk of such force or motion contributing to damage, and therefore much less likelihood of your developing osteoarthritis or aggravating it if it already exists.

You derive another important benefit from correctly aligning your body to deal with force. Correct biomechanical alignment allows you to make the most of your body's power so that, even if you are not particularly strong, you can optimize the strength you do possess and perform feats far beyond your apparent resources. Tiger Woods is neither the strongest pro on the golf circuit nor by any means the heaviest. Yet his body organization is so good that he is able to drive the ball as far as, or farther than, the best of his competitors. He makes the most of his body. Great baseball players of the past like Hank Aaron and Joe DiMaggio had relatively slight frames but made the most of their bodies through brilliantly coordinated and integrated movements. In fact, to this day, Hank Aaron remains the all-time home run king. For all their powerful musculature, today's "pumped up" players have so far been unable to beat Aaron's record.

If you consider the human body as a single unit rather than as a collection of individual "bits," then it follows logically that you have to maintain all of it very carefully. The point is that, over the course of a lifetime, no matter how well we protect ourselves, some small malfunctions are almost bound to arise. And each of these isolated traumas impacts the rest of the body. The effects of these miniassaults build up over time, and if they are not corrected, we soon find ourselves suffering from "bad" backs, knees, etc., and developing osteoarthritis.

Naturally we want to keep our body in balance and operating symmetrically, and therefore subject it to as little wear and tear as possible. Unfortunately, most of us don't know exactly how to do that. Walking, sitting, and standing smoothly and symmetrically, with our center of gravity dead center over our base, is not a natural position. "Stand up straight!" our mothers used to admonish us. "Don't slouch!" But many of us didn't pay attention, and our bad habits persisted. Worse, we usually are not aware of what we're doing wrong or even that we *are* doing anything wrong. Rather, we tend to do what "feels right" without much regard for the long-term implications of our movements. Unfortunately, something feels right because we are used to it—not because it *is* right.

It follows then that almost all of us could use a biomechanical tune-up to counteract the stressful habits we have developed. Chances are that we sit, sleep, lift, drive, type, throw, or otherwise use our bodies in less than perfectly balanced ways. However, since every body is unique, there is no single, comprehensive set of mechanical rules by which we should all live.

Ideally, each one of us should visit a specialist in biomechanics in order to obtain a complete analytic evaluation of how we move. Experts capable of doing this are found among physical therapists, Feldenkrais instructors, tai chi, yoga, and Rolfing instructors, in the ranks of those osteopathic physicians who are board certified in osteopathic manipulative medicine, a few physicians (mainly in sports medicine), and some chiropractors (at the academic level). We should warn you, however, that even within these professions, only a minority of practitioners truly understand biomechanics. Once you understand what you are looking for in a relationship with a practitioner of this type, you will have to interview candidates carefully. Contacting the American Academy of Osteopathy in Indianapolis, Indiana at (317) 879-1881, is one good way of obtaining a referral.

Notwithstanding the fact, which we can never afford to neglect, that every individual is somewhat different, there are nevertheless certain basic biomechanical exercises that can help virtually everyone. And we provide you with a program incorporating the best of them later in this chapter. Before getting into the program, however, we suggest some biomechanical tips and techniques that can help everyone interested in delaying or alleviating osteoarthritis.

Basic Biomechanical Tips and Techniques

Here are some standard approaches to reducing unnecessary stress on your joints while doing everyday activities. Remember, the main principle is to distribute the forces of movement in an even manner to avoid relative overuse—and further joint damage.

Proper Lifting

The force on your lower back increases exponentially as you move an object away from your body. Therefore, always bend your knees when lifting, keeping your back straight and the object you're lifting close to your body. This approach shifts much of the load to the larger and stronger muscles in the legs and buttocks, rather than making your smaller back muscles do all the work.

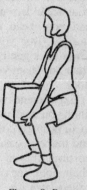

Figure 3. Proper Lifting

Sitting Down

We get in and out of chairs all day long without thinking about the potential for damage that results from our being temporarily out of alignment. To remain aligned—and to avoid placing extra force on some of your vertebrae or on part of your hip joints—use the following simple procedure (it's much easier to do than it is to explain!). To sit, stand tall in front of the chair, feet shoulder-width apart. Place one foot so that the back of that leg is just barely touching the chair, with the other foot very slightly forward. Tighten your abdominal muscles as you bend your knees and push your hips back. Keeping your back straight, moving down and never bending forward, use your leg muscles to ease yourself down into the chair. If the chair has arms, you can hold onto them as you sit. But don't reach down too soon. You want your leg muscles to do most of the work of lowering your body onto the chair.

Sitting

For many people, slouching is the most comfortable sitting position, but that's only because they haven't yet developed their "sitting muscles." Rather than letting go of all muscle tension and sinking into a chair, keep your abdominal muscles gently tight, your shoulders up and slightly back, and your head and neck positioned straight over your spine. Push your lower back gently into the back of the chair and plant your feet firmly on the floor.

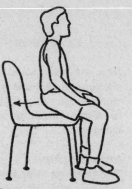

Figure 4. Sitting Down

Experiment with different chairs until you find one that "helps" you to sit properly, one that fits your body and makes it easier to maintain proper posture. If you are using an office chair, look for one that has a feature called *knee tilt*. This allows the back part of your seat to drop down (to rock backward) slightly without the front edge of the chair actually changing in height. The knee tilt feature

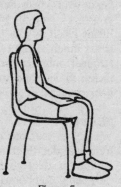

Figure 5.

helps prevent slouching and allows your body weight to be distributed more evenly between your back and your bottom.

The height of the chair is important too. When you are sitting with both feet planted firmly on the floor (don't sit at the desk all day with your legs crossed), your lower leg and thigh should form a right angle. If the chair is too high, you can put a dictionary on the floor and rest your feet on it.

Think about your desk as well. If it's too high, you may be

straining your shoulders as you work. You may need a slightly lower desk (or you could saw down the legs on the one you're using). If the chair has armrests, they should be at a height where your shoulders are in a relaxed position when you are resting your elbows on the armrests. You should not have to elevate or drop your shoulders to reach the arm rests comfortably.

Standing Up

This should be exactly the reverse of sitting down. So rather than throwing your upper body forward, bending severely at the waist, and pushing down on your knees with your hands as you rise, first wiggle or slide yourself to the front of the chair. Both feet should be on the floor near the front of the chair, one slightly forward of the other. Then, keeping your back straight, use your leg muscles to push yourself straight up from the chair. If the chair has arms, press down on the arms with your hands for assistance as you rise. (If the chair has no arms, this approach will also help strengthen your leg muscles, a welcome side effect.)

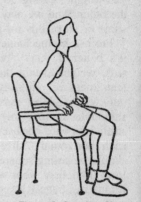

Figure 6. Standing Up

As you can see, the key in sitting down, sitting, and standing up is to keep your back comfortably straight, so that it can support and disperse weight properly. When your back is not comfortably straight, too much force can be exerted on too small a point, such as your lower back. The unfortunate result can be severe pain and permanent injury.

Standing

We've all been standing since we were toddlers, but there's a fair chance that we're doing it improperly, with our backs swayed, shoulders slumped, knees locked, feet askew, belly hanging loose, and weight bearing down on one hip or the other. And we may have been doing some or all of this for a long time.

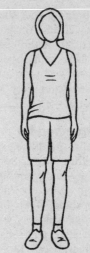

From a biomechanical point of view, it's better if you "stand tall" but not stiff, weight evenly distributed on both feet, knees very slightly bent, abdominal muscles slightly tensed. Your back should be comfortably straight, neither shifted forward nor back. In other words, each horizontal "slice" of your body should be sitting squarely on the one below. Obviously, your weight is now distributed as evenly as possible.

Figure 7. Standing

If you're going to be standing for a few minutes, subtly and slightly shift your weight from one foot to the other every once in a while. Don't push all your weight onto one foot; just shift a little of the burden back and forth. If you're going to be standing for quite a long time, perhaps while ironing, washing dishes, or standing at a bar, lift one foot several inches off the ground and set it on a box or book (or the rail that runs along the bottom of most bars). Shift back and forth so that first one foot, then the other is elevated a few inches. This helps to relieve strain on the lower back.

Holding your stomach in while stand-

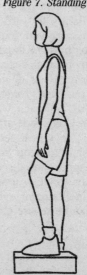

Figure 8. Standing with One Leg Raised

ing is very important because a protruding belly throws off your center of gravity and puts additional strain on your back. This is probably the most important reason that stomach exercises (described in Chapter 5) are so important.

Talking on the Phone

As we talk on the phone, many of us hold the receiver against our shoulders with tilted heads. This is a practical approach because it keeps our hands free, but when overused it can disrupt the biomechanics of the neck. Instead, hold your head up while talking on the phone. Bring the receiver up to your ear instead of dropping your ear to the receiver.

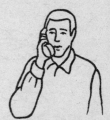

Figure 9. Talking on the Phone

If you need to keep your hands free for writing, you can buy one of the inexpensive telephone headsets at a computer or electronics store.

Sleeping

Overly soft and overly hard mattresses and poor sleeping postures have knocked many spines out of biomechanical balance. Choose a mattress that is firm enough to keep your spine from curving when sleeping on your back or side but has a soft, cushioning *surface* so that your hips can sink in slightly.

A good mattress test is to lie on your side and have someone look at the alignment of your spine while viewing you from the back. Your spine will be curved if the bed is too soft or too hard. One caveat: If your partner is much heavier or lighter than you are, you may have to compromise on mattress firmness to accommodate your differences. If your weights are not too different, you can do this by choosing a mattress that is halfway between your needs. However, if your weights are very different, you may need two single mattresses of different firmnesses placed side by side on a larger box spring.

After several years of use, even the perfect mattress will wear and soften. To stretch its life, rotate and flip your mattress every three months or so to allow it to wear evenly. Then replace it if it can no longer pass the mattress test. The average mattress lasts six to ten years.

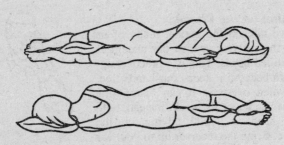

Figure 10. Sleeping

Most biomechanics experts recommend sleeping on your side. You may want to put a pillow between your knees to help reduce stress and increase your comfort. A body pillow (generally five to six feet long) can also support both your lower and upper body. Place the body pillow parallel to you on the side of the bed. Lie on your side facing the pillow and wrap your arm and leg over it. This removes the weight of your arm and leg from the side you are lying on. This can be a great help for people with back, hip, or shoulder arthritis since it can *unload* the affected areas.

If you sleep on your back, consider placing a small pillow underneath your knees. Slightly elevating your knees keeps your back flat. Try to avoid sleeping on your stomach; this can lead to pressure and muscle tightness in your lower back.

Arising from Bed

When arising from bed, most people lift the upper body from a prone to a sitting position on the bed. Then they throw their legs over the side of the bed and haul themselves up. Instead, try this: Wiggle yourself on your side over to the edge of the bed. Then use your arms to push your upper body up while at the same time lowering your legs off the bed. This way, the weight of your legs acts as a counterbalance to help pull the rest of your body up, and your spine stays straight. The result is that there is almost no strain on your lower back. (Try it; it's a very simple habit to adopt, much easier than it sounds on paper.) Once you're sitting on the edge of the bed, use the proper rising technique to stand up. You'll find that getting up from bed in this way is a whole lot easier, especially if you're feeling a bit groggy.

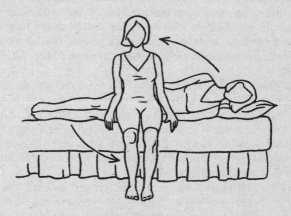

Figure 11. Rising from Bed

If you follow these eight simple tips, you will be astonished by how much easier and less painful everyday tasks become. Moreover, if you don't yet have arthritis in all your joints, then, with virtually no effort you will be helping to delay the onset of the disease in these areas to an impressive extent.

The Biomechanical Program to Increase Your Body's Flexibility

The next step in achieving biomechanical excellence is only slightly more difficult. It consists of building your body's sense of balance—and that is achieved largely by increasing its flexibility.

Proper flexibility is the cornerstone of good biomechanics and is also the cornerstone of our program to maximize your biomechanical behaviors. You may not think that the ability to bend over and touch your toes can help with osteoarthritis, but it can. Good flexibility is important for your joints. Inflexibility in any part of the body exerts extra stress on other areas. This in turn upsets biomechanics, leading to over-compensation, joint stress, and osteoarthritis. Inflexibility can also discourage you from using certain joints. And when you do use those inflexible joints—as you will probably be forced to do from time to time—you are at greater risk of a sprain or strain, because inflexible tissues are more likely to tear or break.

Similarly, agility and balance, which are closely aligned to flexibility, do not directly affect joints, but they do play an important role in joint health. With good agility and balance you are more likely to move about, exercise, and participate in sports—and to keep doing so year after year. This in turn keeps joints well lubricated, keeps extra weight off, and helps keep you healthy all around.

With a platform of flexibility, agility, and balance, you are in a far better position to control your movements correctly, achieve greater results in strength training, and ultimately participate safely in even vigorous physical activities.

In the following pages, we provide you with a program of basic stretches. Please remember, however, that people vary greatly in their degrees of flexibility, so don't worry if you cannot do the full stretch; you are gaining the full benefit from the exercise as long as you are stretching to the limit of *your* capacity. As you keep doing these stretches, you will gradually improve your flexibility. And that's all you should be after: gradual improvement.

Stretching

Simple and easy to do, stretching is a vital part of a biomechanical exercise program. Whether you're training for the

Olympics, combating osteoarthritis, or just trying to stay in shape, *you must stretch regularly.*

Unfortunately, most people don't stretch enough, thinking that jogging or weight lifting are the "real" exercises because that's when they huff and puff and sweat a lot. Moreover, we don't see results from stretching in the form of bigger muscles or faster lap times. And there may not be as much satisfaction in being able to stretch an inch or two farther. Nevertheless, stretching is vital because it keeps us supple and prepares us for lifting those weights and running around that track without harming our muscles or ligaments. Best of all, by counteracting the natural tendency to become stiffer and more sedentary as we age, stretching helps to keep us feeling young, vigorous, and able.

Rules for Successfully Implementing Our Program

Slow and steady is the most important rule. A thirty-second stretch can be significantly more effective than one held for fifteen seconds or less. Here are some other important principles you should follow whenever you stretch.

- Always warm up before stretching. You'll become more flexible more quickly if you warm your muscles before stretching them. Five minutes of moderate activity, or even a warm shower, is sufficient to warm your muscles.
- Relax while moving into a stretch, relax while you're in the stretch, and relax as you release. Remembering to breathe deeply and consistently will help you to achieve this.
- Exhale as you move into a stretch, then continue to breathe steadily.
- Never bounce while stretching; ease into position and hold yourself there.
- Ease into each stretch until you feel mild tension—if you feel pain, you've gone too far. A muscle that is in spasm resists being stretched, and you may injure yourself if you force it.
- Feel the muscular tension draining away from the area you're working as you hold the stretch. If it doesn't, you've gone too far, so ease up a bit.

- Never overstretch. If you can't grab your toes, touch your nose to the floor, or perform a split, don't worry. Instead, focus on doing each stretch properly, slowly becoming more flexible.
- No grimacing allowed! If a stretch is so difficult that you're making unpleasant faces, it hurts, makes you afraid of falling, or has you breathing hard, don't do it. Either this stretch is not for you, or your technique still needs improvement.
- Begin stretching on your "tighter" side. For example, if your left arm is more flexible than your right, stretch your right arm before your left. Most people spend more time on the first limb they stretch, giving shorter shrift to the second. That's why it's helpful to begin with the tighter one. If the discrepancy is great, consider stretching the tight side again after completing the more flexible limb.
- Focus on form when stretching. If your form is good and you stretch diligently, you'll soon be able to reach much farther than you thought possible.
- Remember that flexibility is not constant: Some days you may feel looser than others, depending on what exercises and sports you've been doing or whether you've been sitting all day. Don't worry if you're a little tight one day and can't stretch as far as you could the day before. Instead of overstretching and risking injury, stick with a comfortable stretch and maintain good form. You'll soon regain your temporarily lost flexibility.
- If stretching makes you hurt or feel sick, stop and see your physician to make sure you are not suffering from heart problems or any disease.
- Know which areas of your body are supposed to be enhanced by each stretch. If you don't feel the mild tension in the correct area as you do each stretch, you may be doing it improperly.

Keep these principles in mind when beginning our stretching program, which starts with the large muscles in your legs, then moves up to your hips, back, and neck. (Again, consult your physician before starting any new exercise regimen.) The program is simple and can be done in a limited amount of

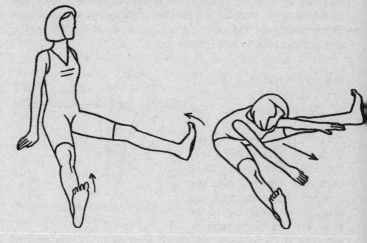

Figure 12. Hamstring Stretch

time. But if you do it all, you'll have completed a total-body stretch in 20–30 minutes. And you'll feel terrific!

HAMSTRING STRETCH

First, seat yourself comfortably on a cushioned floor or exercise mat. Do this by lowering one knee to the floor then your other knee, keeping your body straight as you do so. Next, place one arm on the ground, bending your upper body as necessary, and lower yourself to a seated position. Stretch your legs in a V, keeping your knees as straight as you can and your toes flexed upward. Try to keep your back straight and your chin up. Carefully inch your whole trunk forward between your legs until you feel a strain in the back of your legs. Hold the stretch for thirty seconds. Then, while tightening your abdominals, sit back up and rest for fifteen seconds. Bend down again, holding it for another thirty seconds. Exhale as you try to move down farther. Do not cheat by allowing your knees to bend; this will make your stretch relatively ineffective. (Figure 12 shows the woman touching the floor. You may not be able to do that. But, to repeat, that's not the important part. As long as you feel the stretch in your hamstrings and behind your knees, it's working. And eventually maybe you *will* be able to touch your toes.)

ISOLATED HAMSTRING STRETCH
This exercise is an extension of the previous one. Flex your toes and keep your knees perfectly straight. With your back straight, lean forward from your trunk over your right leg, reaching forward with your chest and arms toward your right foot. Stay there for thirty seconds,

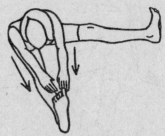

Figure 13. Isolated Hamstring Stretch

exhaling as you deepen the stretch. Rest for thirty seconds and repeat once. Do the same exercise with your left leg.

PROPRIOCEPTIVE NEUROMUSCULAR FACILITATION
Proprioceptive neuromuscular facilitation (or PNF) is a technique that lets you "uncouple" the stretch reflexes that normally keep you from injuring yourself. Normally, when you stretch, your muscles automatically "clench" to avoid stretching too far. You can do this without fear of injury because you're resting comfortably on the ground, so that uncoupling your protective stretch reflexes is safe. Contract the muscle that you're trying to stretch for five to eight seconds, and then relax it, breathing out as you do so (which helps you relax). Doing this enables you to stretch farther than you normally can.

In these first exercises, try implementing PNF between your first and second stretch on each side. Keep your knees straight and try to push one or both of your heels into the ground, thus contracting the hamstring muscles. Hold the contraction for five to eight seconds. Relax. After doing this, in your second stretch you should be able to reach a little bit farther.

PNF works on virtually all types of stretches. So once you have the idea, try it between repetitions every time you stretch.

BUTTERFLY STRETCH

This stretch improves the external rotation of your hips. Sit with your back against a wall and the soles of your feet together. Then, while loosely holding your ankles, bend forward from your lower back, chest and abs tight. Using your elbows to help push

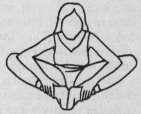

Figure 14. Butterfly Stretch

your knees down, relax your legs as much as possible. Hold that position for about thirty seconds. Using your abdominals, return to your original seating position. Rest for thirty seconds, then repeat.

You can do PNF here, squeezing your legs toward the ceiling, while pushing them down with your arms. Hold that tension for five to eight seconds. Relax and breathe. As you exhale, repeat the stretch; it should improve.

ARROW STRETCH

This stretch is for the sides of your buttocks, hips, and outsides of your thighs. The arrow stretch is a powerful tool used as both a treatment and prevention of several orthopedic problems, including hip bursitis, problems with alignment of the kneecaps, and ITB syndrome, the most common running injury. ITB stands for iliotibial band, a long piece of fibrous connective tissue that runs on the outside of your hip and thigh all the way down from the crest of your hip to just below the knee. If the ITB is too tight, it can rub on the hip and cause bursitis. Or it can pull on the kneecap, leading to malalignment and pain. When the iliotibial band rubs the side of the knee, the resultant pain is called ITB syndrome. Stretching creates some slack in the ITB and can help with all of these problems.

Note: Osteoarthritis and hip bursitis are often confused. Therefore, it is worth knowing the difference before you start stretching. To tell, feel the outside of your hip where the bony part sticks out. With your fingertips, gently but firmly push the area right over the bone. If that causes you pain, it's likely due to bursitis. If you feel you have bursitis, talk to your doctor. Bursitis is a very different condition, with different treatments, from osteoarthritis.

Start the arrow stretch by lying on your side. Bend the knee closer to the ground and bring it toward your chest. Keep the other leg relatively straight (but do not lock the knee). The stretch gets its name from the "arrow" your legs form when you're in this position.

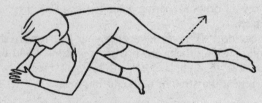

Figure 15. Arrow Stretch

Now try to bring your trunk and head, aligned, directly over your knee, and touch your forehead to the ground. Unless you're very limber, you won't get all the way there, but you should feel a stretch on the outside of your hip and buttocks on the side closer to the ground. If you don't feel a stretch, adjust the position of your hips so they are facing more parallel to the ground, and less sideways. This increases the stretch. Hold for thirty seconds. Relax and repeat. Then do the same procedure on your other side.

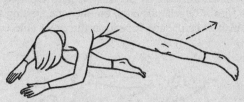

Figure 16. Arrow Stretch

LEG PULL

This is a comfortable way to stretch a difficult area, the front of your thigh. It's best to do this after you have done the other leg and hip stretches described above. Lie on your right side. Bring your left knee forward so that its side touches the ground at the level of your waist. Bend your right knee, keeping your body in a straight line through the trunk, and reach down with your left hand and grab your right ankle. Extend your right hip so that you feel a stretch along the front of your thigh. Now, gently pull your ankle closer to your buttocks to increase the stretch in this area. Do not twist the knee; keep your leg aligned. Hold for thirty seconds or more, then switch sides, repeating the procedure with the opposite hand and leg.

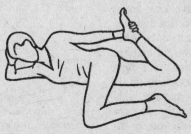

Figure 17. Leg Pull

If this stretch becomes too easy, and your foot easily reaches your buttocks, put a cushion under the front part of the leg you are stretching and position your knee so that it's facing down toward the ground. This extends the hip farther and makes it more difficult to do this stretch. Do two of these stretches for thirty seconds each on one side, resting for a few seconds in between. Then repeat on the other side.

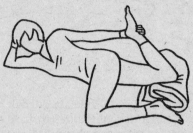

Figure 18. Leg Pull

You can do this stretch even if your knee doesn't bend all the way due to arthritis. As long as your hip is okay, you can extend your hip and still stretch your quadriceps (thigh muscles) and hip flexors without having to grasp your ankle and/or bend your knee too far.

DOUBLE HIP ROTATION
This stretch is difficult to do unless you have long arms. Also, it's important that you do this stretch only after you've done the leg and hip stretches so that your hips are properly loosened up. If you cannot manage this stretch alone, try to get someone to help you, or do one leg at a time.

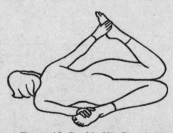

Figure 19. Double Hip Rotation

To appreciate the benefit of this stretch, you need to understand that your hips move in six directions: forward and back, inward and outward, and in clockwise or counterclockwise rotation. The first four of these motions are routine and require no extra stretching. However, the rotational movements, called internal hip rotations, are rarely performed and little mentioned in most stretching instruction manuals. They are important, however, because loss of internal hip rotation may lead to osteoarthritis in the lower back years later.

To perform this stretch, lie on your stomach, spreading your legs a comfortable width apart. Then bend your knees to a 90-degree angle. Reach behind you and gently grab your ankles or feet with your hands. Gently push your feet apart until you feel the stretch. Be sure to keep your knees together as you do this; there's a tendency for them to separate as you move farther into the stretch. Hold the stretch for fifteen to thirty seconds, rest, and repeat once.

REACHING CROSSOVER

This is a great stretch for your back and spine. Lie flat on your back with your arms at your sides. Bend your left leg and lift it up and in toward your chest. Next, still bent, cross that leg over your right leg (which is still stretched straight). Keeping your trunk flat with both shoulders on the ground, reach above and slightly to the left with both arms.

Hold the stretch for ten seconds, relax, and repeat once or twice. Then do the same on the other side, reversing the direction in which you stretch your arms. Don't be surprised if you temporarily feel a little taller after doing this one!

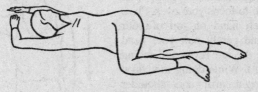

Figure 20. Reaching Crossover

NECK STRETCH

The final two exercises stretch your neck muscles. First, sit upright in a chair, your head turned just slightly to the left. Gently move your head down and slightly to the right with

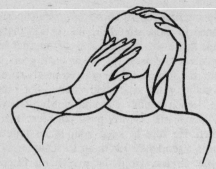

Figure 21. Neck Stretch 1

your right hand. With your left hand, push on the tendons where your neck extensor muscles emerge from your skull. Tenderness in these tendons resolves over time. If you get tension headaches, this may help lessen their severity or even prevent them. You can also turn your head to varying degrees, first ten degrees, then try it at twenty degrees, and then maybe even thirty. Repeat the stretch, then turn your head to the right and use the opposite hand to perform the stretch on the other side. Spend thirty to sixty seconds on each side.

NECK STRETCH
Again, sit in a chair. While looking straight ahead, pick a spot on
the wall to focus your eyes. Place
your left hand on top of your
head and gently pull your head
toward the left (eyes still facing
the spot). While doing this, drop
your right arm and shoulder
down, and reach gently downward as if you were reaching for
something on the ground. You'll
feel a gentle pull on the muscle

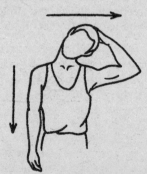

Figure 22. Neck Stretch 2

on the right side of the neck. Hold for thirty to sixty seconds. Repeat the procedure on the other side with the opposite hand.

We urge you to complete this program in full every day. It doesn't take much time, less than half an hour, and it doesn't take much effort. It will greatly improve your flexibility and will help treat your osteoarthritis joints and may even reduce your chances of developing any in places where it hasn't yet struck.

Supplemental Exercises to Improve Flexibility Once You've Mastered the Basic Program

As you follow the above program, you will stretch most large muscle groups in your body. However, after a while, you may find that there are certain places you are not reaching with these stretches. Now that the rest of you is looser, you may realize that these trouble spots could also stand some loosening up. So here is a supplemental set of exercises. Choose the ones that are right for you and slowly build them into the basic program described in the previous section.

We discuss these important stretches in descending order from the top of the body on down, starting with the neck and shoulders and finishing with the ankles and feet.

NECK AND SHOULDERS

NECK BEND AND TWIST

You can stand or sit for this stretch, but sitting feels a little more comfortable to most people. Drop your head down toward your chest and hold it there for ten seconds. Lift your head, then lower it to the left, moving your left ear down toward your left shoulder, and hold it there for ten seconds. Lift your head, then lower it to the right, moving your right ear down toward your right shoulder, and hold it there for ten seconds. Now lift your head and turn it to the left as if you were looking at someone standing over your left shoulder, and hold it there for ten seconds. Repeat the stretch by turning your head to the right and hold the stretch for ten seconds.

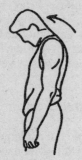
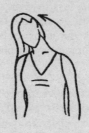
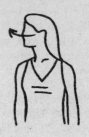

Figure 23. Neck Bend and Twist

SHOULDER CIRCLES

Stand comfortably straight with your
feet slightly apart. With your arms
hanging at your sides, lift your shoulders up, forward, down, back, up, and
forward to complete a shoulder circle.
Make those circles as smooth as possible, and repeat them ten times. Then
do ten reverse shoulder circles (up,
back, down, forward, up, and back).
Finish by lifting your shoulders up as
far as they go, holding them in place
for ten seconds, then gently dropping
them back down to their normal position.

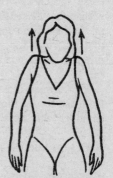

*Figure 24. Shoulder
Circles*

ARM PULL

Stand comfortably straight, with your
feet slightly apart. Tilt your head
slightly down and toward your left
shoulder, and hold for thirty seconds.
Reach both hands behind your back.
Grasp your right hand with your left

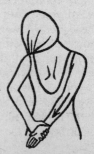

Figure 25. Arm Pull

and gently pull your right arm diagonally across your back toward your left buttock. Hold for thirty seconds. Repeat stretch on the other side.

ARMS

WRAPAROUND

Either sit or stand comfortably upright. Put your right hand on your left shoulder. With your left hand on your right arm above the elbow, push your right arm toward your left shoulder until you feel a comfortable stretch in the back of your right shoulder and upper arm. Hold for thirty seconds. Repeat on the other side.

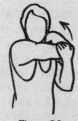

Figure 26.
Wraparound

OVERHEAD SHOULDER PULL

Stand comfortably straight with your feet slightly apart and your knees slightly bent. Put your right arm over the top of your head (so your right fingers are pointing down toward your left shoulder). Grasp above your right elbow with your left hand and gently pull your arm across and down to the left. You may have to tilt your head forward slightly to get it out of the way. Gently and carefully continue the stretch, then deepen it by bending from your waist to the left until you feel a comfortable stretch along your entire right side, from your armpit to the bottom of your hip. Hold for thirty seconds. Repeat on the other side.

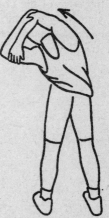

Figure 27. Overhead
Shoulder Pull

ARMS UP

Stand comfortably straight with your
feet slightly apart and your knees
slightly bent. Hold a towel by the
ends behind your neck. Straighten
your arms and lift them up and behind
you until you feel a comfortable
stretch. Hold the stretch for thirty seconds, then gently lower your arms.

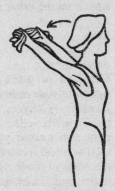

Figure 28. Arms Up

A variation of this exercise can really help stretch the thoracic spine
(midback), normally a difficult area to
reach. Sit in an office chair with a
firm but padded back. The top of the
chair's back should reach to about the
level of your shoulder blades, no
higher. Reach back as you would in the standing exercise. The
top edge of the chair will push the thoracic spine forward as
your body weight is shifted backward. This is a form of *self-
manipulation* of the spine.

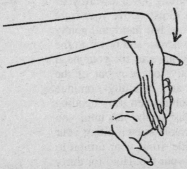

Figure 29. Wrist-Fingers Stretch—Flexion

Hands, Fingers, Wrists

WRIST-FINGERS STRETCH—FLEXION

Either standing or sitting comfortably straight, hold your arms out in front of you, with your elbows straight. Turn your right palm up. With your left hand, gently pull back the tips of your fingers. Hold for thirty seconds. Be sure to keep your right elbow straight. Repeat on the other side.

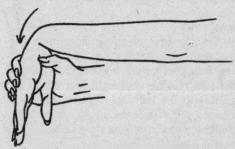

Figure 30. Wrist Stretch—Extension

WRIST STRETCH—EXTENSION

Either standing or sitting comfortably straight, hold your arms out in front of you, with your elbows straight. Turn your left palm down. Place the fingertips of your right hand just above the knuckles of your left hand. Relax your left hand and gently pull it back and down, using your right hand. Hold for thirty seconds. Be sure to keep your right elbow straight. Repeat on the other side.

Back

LOOK BEHIND

Standing comfortably straight with your hands on your hips, gently twist at the waist, turning back toward the right until you feel a comfortable stretch in your back. Twist back to center then around to the left to complete a single look behind. Repeat a total of three times.

If you prefer, you can do this stretch with a pole (say, a broomstick) resting on your neck behind your head and your arms holding the ends of the pole. That way, you can comfortably swing back and forth farther because you get more torque. Keep your knees slightly bent when you do this to avoid placing any twisting motion on them.

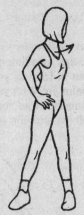

Figure 31. Look Behind

SITTING TRUNK TWIST

Sitting comfortably straight on the floor or your mat, extend your left leg straight out to the front. Bend your right leg and cross it over your left, placing your right foot on the ground just to the outside of your left knee. Bend your left arm at the elbow, then place your elbow outside of your right knee. Put your right hand flat on the floor, slightly behind your right hip. Now turn your head to the right and press your left elbow into your right knee as you twist back and around to the right. Balance your weight on your buttocks—try to keep both cheeks on the floor—and

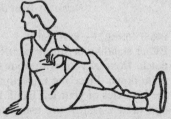

Figure 32. Sitting Trunk Twist

your right hand. Hold for thirty seconds, then repeat on the other side.

GROIN AND INNER THIGHS

SWAY STRETCH

Stand straight with your legs spread slightly farther apart than your shoulders. With your hands on your hips, slightly bend your right knee as you let your left hip gently move downward toward your right knee. Make sure that your bent knee remains in alignment with your ankles, so that your knee is right over the center of your foot. You should feel the stretch in your left inner thigh and groin. Hold the stretch for thirty seconds, then repeat on other side.

KNEE TO CHEST
Lie flat on your back. Using both hands, pull your left knee up to your chest, keeping your other leg flat and flexed until you feel a com-

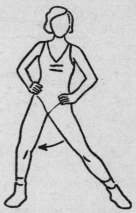

Figure 33. Sway Stretch

fortable stretch. Be sure to pull from under your knee rather than pressing on the kneecap. Hold for thirty seconds. Repeat with other leg.

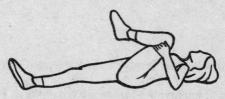

Figure 34. Knee to Chest

ANKLES AND FEET

THE RACK
Lie flat on your back. Raise your arms up over your head and rest them on the floor beyond your head. Now stretch your arms, fingers, legs, feet, and toes. Hold for thirty seconds. Relax. Repeat.

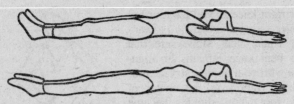

Figure 35. The Rack

FOOT CIRCLES

Stand comfortably straight with your feet together. Resting one hand lightly on the wall or a table for balance, lift your right foot about twelve inches off the ground. Rotate your ankle and foot clockwise ten times, then counterclockwise ten times. Repeat with your left foot.

This exercise also can be done lying flat on your back, as with *the rack,* following the same steps as above.

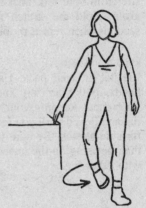

Figure 36. Foot Circles

Exercises to Improve Balance and Agility

In addition to improving your overall flexibility, it is important that you practice achieving biomechanical balance more directly, which is the primary purpose of the following exercises. These are the exercises we recommend for people (most of us) who need to develop additional balance and agility.

Several of these exercises require an inexpensive device that incorporates a waist belt or strap, with rubber tubing, to offer resistance. Several brands, such as Theraband and Proten, exist. They can usually be obtained at a local medical supply store or through a physical therapist's office.

Physical therapists are excellent resources for monitoring

your program and teaching you new exercises once you've mastered this basic program. Ask your physician to prescribe a few visits with a physical therapist since your medical insurance company is unlikely to pay for a self-referral. Fortunately, there are many ways you can improve your biomechanics on your own. So, let's get started.

The first few exercises in this program enhance your ability to transfer weight from one side of your body to the other smoothly and with a minimum of jarring.

Silent Walking

This is best performed with hard-soled shoes on a hard surface so that you can hear the sound of your footsteps. First, walk normally and focus on the sound of your footsteps. Loudness translates into higher force being placed on the joints in the lower body. Now walk while consciously quieting your gait. Try to figure out why your normal gait is so much louder and try to make your body move more fluidly by using your upper and lower body in a rhythmic manner. At first, although you will be able to walk much more quietly, the movement will feel forced. After some practice, however, you will notice that your gait is changing so that, even without concentrating, you are walking more quietly and lowering the impact on your joints.

Practice this exercise for three to five minutes (the length of a typical song on the radio), then move on the next exercise.

Slow Stair Climbing

Most people use momentum to climb stairs. That is, they push off from one leg in order to generate the momentum to raise the other leg to the next stair. Instead, try moving slowly from step to step, with no momentum to push off, only the work of contracting the muscles in the front of your thighs. You may find that initially your legs are too weak to climb slowly, even though you are able to climb stairs at a normal pace. But keep trying to reduce the amount of push-off you need. This exercise can quickly improve your balance and strength; you should notice an improvement within a couple of weeks. One flight of stairs (about fourteen steps) is fine to start with. Soon you'll be doing sets of three. Then, as you become more advanced, try doing the same exercise while climing two steps at a time.

Balancing on One Foot

Standing upright, raise your right leg a foot off the ground, while balancing on your left. Hold this position for thirty seconds, lower your foot to the ground, and repeat on the other side.

Holding in your abdominal muscles will help you keep your balance—really. It may also help you at first to hold your arms out to the side, parallel to the floor. When you can do the exercise without wobbling, try it with your arms crossed. For an advanced challenge, close your eyes while doing the exercise. This is more difficult than it sounds, so be careful.

Tiptoe Balance

Stand upright with your knees straight or slightly bent and raise your right leg off the ground while balancing on your left foot. Now lift your left heel off the ground, balancing on the ball of your foot until you're standing on tiptoe. Hold this position for ten seconds, lower your foot to the ground, and repeat on the other side. At first you may not be able to do this without holding onto something to maintain your balance. But keep trying; after a while your balance will improve.

The next part of the program enhances your agility. It requires you to be functional enough to jog or run short distances (1/4 mile or less). *Note:* these are advanced exercises in biomechanics. You need not do all of them. We suggest that you choose two or three of them during each exercise session and keep rotating them.

Running Figure Eights

Run in figure-eight patterns, starting with a large one and getting progressively smaller. Then run through the figure eights again, backward. You will find you can do this exercise easily only if you are well balanced. The more you practice it—and the better you get at it—the better will be your biomechanical balance. Practice this for about three minutes running forward, and three minutes running backward.

Carioka Step

This part of our program will make sure that you are walking without leaning in one direction or another. For example, if you lean forward when you walk normally, you will notice that you can hardly keep your balance when you do the same thing while walking sideways. You will be forced to correct yourself.

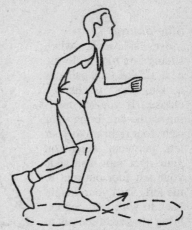

Figure 37. Running Figure Eights

This first exercise requires you to move sideways, crossing one leg in front, then behind. Thus, if you move to the left, your right leg crosses in front of your left. The next step brings you to the starting position, and on the third step you cross your right leg behind your left leg, and so on. Start by doing this exercise at a walk until you get the hang of it, then progress to a run. Practice this for about three minutes going in each direction.

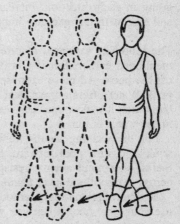

Figure 38. Carioka Step

You can also do this on a treadmill. Set its speed to somewhat slower than a normal walk, then increase the speed gradually as your ability improves.

Side Shuffle

Move sideways, while sliding one foot up to the next. (If you took ballet as a kid, this is like a chassé.) If you are moving to the left, bring your right foot right up to your left, put your weight on your right foot, and slide your left foot out and to the left. Shift your weight back to your left foot and bring your right foot up to the left. Practice this exercise for three minutes

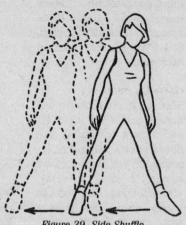

Figure 39. Side Shuffle

going in each direction. Increase your speed, as your agility and ease with this exercise improve.

The following exercises require resistance, the elastic belt we mentioned earlier. But if you don't have the belt, you aren't off the hook. All these exercises can be done in a swimming pool. Water offers a great deal of resistance without harming the joints, it makes you feel weightless, and splashing around in the water is fun.

For the walking against resistance exercise, for example, walk across the pool forward, then walk back backward. For the side stepping against resistance exercise, walk sideways across the pool and back again.

Midmorning and midafternoon are usually the best times to use your local pool, when you won't get in the way of serious swimmers doing laps.

Walking Against Resistance

Place an elasticized strap around your waist then anchor it to the doorknob of a securely closed door. Walk forward several steps until the pressure stops you from proceeding. Walk back to the starting point. Repeat at least ten times forward. Then repeat the exercise ten times while walking backward. As you get more practiced, you can do the exercises jogging—be careful not to move so far that the elastic band yanks you backward like a cartoon character!

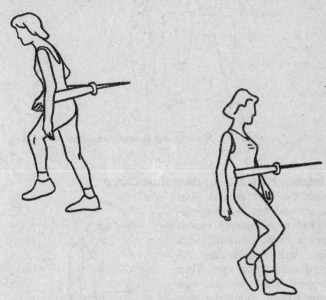

Figure 40. Walking Against Resistance

Sidestepping Against Resistance

With the belt around your waist (and its end securely anchored to a closed door's knob), move several steps sideways, crossing one leg in front of the other as you go. Return to the starting position, crossing the same foot in front. Then turn around and sidestep in the other direction. Repeat at least ten times on each side.

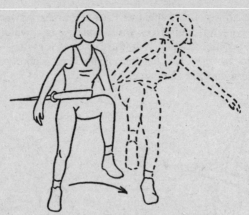

Figure 41. Sidestepping Against Resistance

Lunging Forward Against Resistance

With the belt around your waist, and the belt end anchored to a securely closed door's knob, push off with your right foot, lunging forward onto your left. Your forward foot, the one you lunged onto, should be bent at no more than a 90-degree angle, that is, your knee should not be forward of your ankle. Return to starting position and lunge forward onto the other foot. Repeat at least ten times for each leg. This is an exercise where, again, you must be careful to

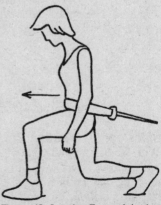

Figure 42. Lunging Forward Against Resistance

use your muscles and not momentum to execute properly.

Lunges are good for stretching your thighs and for building their strength. However, they also build balance, especially when you use a resistance belt. It's hard to explain exactly how this works, but try it for yourself with and without a belt, and you'll see what we mean.

Lunging Sideways
Against Resistance

This exercise is similar to the forward lunge described previously, but this time stand with the belt around your waist, your right side facing out from the wall. Squat so that your knees are bent at about a 90-degree angle. Push off with your left leg and lunge out to the right. Then push off with your right leg to return to the starting position. Repeat at least ten times. Then turn around and lunge sideways with your left side facing out and repeat ten more times.

Now you have a complete yet simple biomechanics program. If you do it regularly (at least three times per week), your biomechanics will improve dramatically—and you will feel great. The following worksheet will help you to put together your own program, and keep you on track once you've started. Make copies of the worksheet and plaster them on the fridge to monitor your progress.

Popular Alternative Approaches to Bettering Biomechanics

There are many other ways of improving your biomechanical balance. Some are fun to do just in themselves. Several have additional advantages aside from improving your biomechanics. Thus, while many traditional Western physicians don't acknowledge that these alternative bodywork therapies have value, many people have been helped by Feldenkrais, Rolfing, tai chi, yoga, and other techniques.

But there are pitfalls. Unlike medical doctors, osteopathic physicians, chiropractors, and physical therapists, all of whom go through carefully prescribed and regulated training and licensing procedures, alternative therapists have varying degrees

BIOMECHANICS PROGRESS CHART

	EXERCISES		MON.	TUES.	WED.	THURS.	FRI.	SAT.	SUN.
Biomechanical Stretching	Basic Program (to be done every day)	Hamstring Stretch							
		Isolated Hamstring Stretch							
		Butterfly Stretch							
		Arrow Stretch							
		Leg Pull							
		Double Hip Rotation							
		Reaching Crossover							
		Neck Stretch 1							
		Neck Stretch 2							
	Supplemental Exercises for Stiff Spots (can be done every day)	Neck/Shoulders — Bend/Twist							
		Neck/Shoulders — Shoulder Circles							
		Neck/Shoulders — Arm Pull							
		Arms — Wraparound							
		Arms — Overhead Pull							
		Arms — Arms Up							
		Hands, Fingers, Wrist — W-F Stretch							
		Hands, Fingers, Wrist — Wrist Stretch							
		Back — Look Behind							
		Back — Sitting Trunk Twist							
		Groin and Thigh — Sway Stretch							
		Groin and Thigh — Knee to Chest							
		Ankles and Feet — The Rock							
		Ankles and Feet — Foot Circles							

Improving Balance and Agility (select at least two from each category, rotating regularly)	Balance	Silent Walking									
		Slow Stair Climbing									
		Balance on One Foot									
		Tiptoe Balance									
	Agility	Running Figure Eights									
		Carioka Step									
		Side Shuffle									
		Walking Against Resistance									
		Sidestepping Against Resistance									
		Lunging Forward Against Resistance									
		Lunging Sideways Against Resistance									

Check the box when you do the exercise.

of education, practical training, and skill. Some have gone through extensive preparation, others have not, and the approaches they espouse range from the valuable to the absurd. So be careful in choosing the techniques and practitioners. Interview instructors about their background. Don't be afraid to ask where they got their training and for how long. Also ask for references from past clients; if they won't respond promptly and openly, move on. Also, you may want to contact the organization or school that certified or accredited the practitioner to check on how much training was required to earn a certificate or other accreditation.

Nothing can take the place of your own common sense and good judgment. However, a little up-front knowledge may help you, so here are descriptions of some practices you may find useful.

The Feldenkrais Method

During the early part of this century, a young Polish boy named Moshe Feldenkrais injured his knee while playing soccer. Years later, during World War II, he found himself practically living aboard a ship to conduct antisubmarine research for the British Navy.

The constant pitching of the boat aggravated the old injury. A prominent physician offered to perform surgery. He warned that, while he could only offer a 50 percent chance of success, there was a 100 percent certainty that, if the surgery were not performed soon, the knee would degenerate irreparably. Faced with such an unpalatable choice, Feldenkrais decided to find—or devise—a therapy that would cure his knee without the risk of surgery. Following a comprehensive study of physiology, anatomy, kinesiology, yoga, and other disciplines, he developed his own system later to become known as the Feldenkrais method.

Feldenkrais training is designed to reeducate mind and body as you develop new, more healthy and efficient ways of moving. It's felt that we learn our original, perhaps unhealthy, ways of walking, sitting, throwing a ball, etc., by "watching and doing" when we are very young, and these movement patterns are imprinted in the circuitry of our central nervous systems. Thus, Feldenkrais theorized, we should also learn new, healthy methods by watching and doing, not by talking or studying diagrams. And we should continue to practice until the new techniques replace the old in our mental circuitry so that the new ways feel natural.

During the first part of Feldenkrais training, called *functional integration,* practitioners use their hands to guide body parts through the proper movements. As these movements are performed over and over again, they "imprint" themselves on patients' central nervous systems and become "natural." In the second phrase of training, called *awareness through movement,* the practitioner leads an individual or group of students through a series of movements. But these are not preset movements that must be mirrored perfectly. Instead, students are encouraged to find the variation that's just right for them.

The goal of Feldenkrais training is to teach you to move naturally and freely, without stress or tension. The entire body is to be turned from a rigid "machine" into a flowing organism that slides gently from movement to movement, never generating unneeded muscle stress or unnatural breathing.

Rolfing

Properly known as *structural integration,* Rolfing was developed in the late 1920s to encourage physical, emotional, and spiritual health. Biochemist Ida Rolf based her system on the idea that the human body is made up of several segments (head, shoulders, chest, etc.). Each segment must sit atop the next and be in perfect alignment with all the others for the body to function properly.

When our body segments are misaligned, we cannot move properly, and our strides and motions are hindered and distorted. This can be corrected by manipulating the myofascial tissue, a thin but very elastic tissue linking and connecting the body parts to each other. In this manner, the myofascia and muscles are lengthened and "unstuck," allowing the body segments to move back into proper vertical alignment.

Many people cringe when you mention Rolfing, for they've heard that it's a very painful procedure. It need not hurt. Modern Rolfers have devised less strenuous, more gentle techniques. They have also incorporated muscle and ligament manipulation to help work misaligned joints back into place.

Rolfing takes about ten sessions, each one focusing on a different part of the body. Afterward, you notice that you aren't noticing your body anymore. It moves with greater fluidity and without stress.

Rolfing can be helpful in some cases, and it's hard to see how it could do damage. However, there is very little solid research on the approach. We therefore suggest that you participate in the activity only if, after trying it, you enjoy it and feel it's valuable to you.

Tai Chi Chuan

Although tai chi chuan (pronounced "tie jee chew-on") means "supreme ultimate fist," the art is designed to stimulate quiet and peacefulness in movement. Based on the idea that good health comes from balance and a constant flow of energy, tai chi teaches a series of movements and postures that flow from one to the next, easily and fluidly. The gentle circular and other types of continuous movement exercise muscles all over the body. Rather than completing one posture before moving into the next, the goal is to continually shift body weight, contract and relax muscles, turn from side to side, and rotate body angles. There should not be strain on any part of your body; instead, the aim is to keep your body grounded and aligned. As you learn to move smoothly from one posture to another, your legs become stronger and your body awareness more acute. You also learn to relax while performing difficult maneuvers.

More advanced students practice "pushing hands," learning to move in response to a partner, developing a keener appreciation of body weight, muscle balance, and their own center of gravity.

We have little doubt that this technique improves biomechanical balance. Whether you decide to adopt the technique or not should depend on whether you enjoy it.

Yoga

An ancient system arising in India some five thousand years ago, yoga is an integrated approach to mental, emotional, physical, and spiritual development. The word *yoga* means "union of the self with the divine."

Yoga postures (asanas) can help improve biomechanics while stretching, strengthening, and toning the body. The movements, performed while standing, seated, or lying, are done slowly and thoughtfully. In a properly designed series of postures, every moment "is an exercise in itself with the specific purpose of repairing and maintaining individual parts of your body. However, taking one pose to benefit one alignment is limiting. The purpose of yoga is to benefit the whole body, not just its parts."[1]

There are many schools of yoga, each emphasizing a different part of the ancient art. All, however, use more or less the same postures and breathing exercises. Many Americans have been turned off by yoga because they have heard of the spiritual and religious teachings inherent in some of the traditionally taught yoga classes. When yoga was first introduced into the United States, many yoga instructors did incorporate the full gamut of spiritual teachings into their classes. However, today most yoga instructors focus mainly on the movements themselves and not the religious teachings.

Since there is no "official" school of yoga, you'll find different classes being taught different ways at local schools, gyms, and Ys. The best class for you is the one in which you feel most comfortable, challenged to improve but not pushed beyond your capabilities. Move up to a more difficult level as you progress in your abilities. Yoga is an excellent form of exercise for improving biomechanics in someone with arthritis. It may have preventive value as well.

---

1. A. Finger and L. Guber, *Yoga Moves* (New York: Wallaby Books, 1984), p. 20.

There is no single "correct" approach to developing good biomechanics. That means that you have to do a little research to find the method that is best for you. It also means that, almost certainly, there is a technique out there that perfectly suits your needs.

One emphatic recommendation: Even if you decide not to spend a great deal of time on biomechanics, and you do not find a suitable instructor to help you, do take the limited time it requires to complete, once a day, the basic biomechanical program described and illustrated earlier in this chapter. You and your joints will feel a great deal better!

5

Aerobics and Strength

The pain and suffering of osteoarthritis often cause people to cut down on exercise or even to give it up altogether. That is very understandable and makes intuitive sense. After all, we are taught early on that when a movement hurts, we should refrain from it.

For short periods, this advice really does make sense. Our bodies need to recuperate after heavy activity or training. But prolonged inactivity (more than one to two weeks) is bad for you. In the long run, it leads to secondary problems, including loss of muscle tone, muscle weakness, joint contracture, lack of endurance, and poor body mechanics. In effect, your muscles and joints will "shrink and stiffen up," making normal movement harder. When these problems settle in, it hurts more than ever to move, increasing your desire to do nothing while driving up the odds of reinjury whenever you are forced into some activity.

If you have osteoarthritis and you want to get better, you *must* exercise. Of course, you need to tailor your exercise to your level of ability, starting slowly and gradually increasing. Exercise should never hurt you. It should push you to the edge of pain but not over it. That is what this chapter is about: how to start an antiosteoarthritis exercise program that feels good, gradually increases the flexibility of your joints by driving synovial fluid into them, strengthens your muscles, improves your endurance and energy, and thus maximizes the impact of the arthritis cure.

Exercise by itself cannot cure osteoarthritis. It can, however, solve many of the potentially painful and dangerous secondary problems associated with the disease. Remember, when the muscles around a joint are toned and strong, your joints are stabilized better, so that pressure placed on them as you move about does them less harm. Thus, exercise can greatly ease long-term pain, improve your general health, help you manage your daily tasks better, speed your return to the activities you enjoy, and improve your outlook on life.

First, let us give you a general tip about exercise that will help you adopt the right attitude to the program we set forth in this chapter: Instead of measuring the value of your exercise program by the level of your pain, think about the pleasure you are gaining from improving your ability to handle life's tasks. The point is that if you keep thinking about how much pain you have, *you will feel it more*. Instead, choose some positive, objective criteria to keep track of your improvement. Can you walk farther than before? Can you get a hold of the things that you were unable to reach or grasp before? Can you lift heavier objects? Are you able to perform routine tasks that you used to avoid? Can you handle more of your self-care? Have you returned to some recreational or sports activities you had to avoid in the past? Are you taking less pain medicine? If the answer to any of these questions is yes, your exercise program is helping.

Of course, you do not want to do exercises that osteoarthritis makes especially uncomfortable or painful. There is no point in martyring yourself with actions that are just too painful to bear. But rather than giving up on exercise altogether, you need to work *around* the problem. For instance, if you are having knee pain while walking or using a treadmill, consider riding a bicycle or stationary bike instead. Riding jolts your knees much less than running but still gives them exercise. If you are still having problems, you may have to do something simpler, such as leg lifts in a swimming pool or with light ankle weights. The key is not to stop but to modify your activities.

There are numerous benefits to a good exercise program in addition to its help in treating osteoarthritis. Exercise can improve resistance to disease, enhance balance and coordination, reduce stress while improving emotional health, encourage relaxation and induce a good night's sleep, improve body composition by building muscle while burning fat, and even enhance your sex life. Exercise also can help you preserve your independence by building the health and strength you need to continue living on your own.

Unfortunately, our health doesn't "stay put" if we stop exercising. The human body was made to move—if we stop moving, we increase the risk of developing heart disease, obesity, diabetes, high blood pressure, and a bunch of other ailments. Heart disease and cancer are the top two killers in this country today. But the *causes* of these diseases are mostly related to two factors, smoking and a sedentary lifestyle. Fortunately, lack of exercise is a very preventable problem. It is, after all, merely an unfortunate habit. But because it is a habit, you can retrain yourself and begin reversing your behavior today. All it takes is desire and the knowledge of which exercises work best for you.

The Maximizing Exercise Program

There are four basic aspects to fitness that are an essential part of the arthritis cure:

- Flexibility
- Agility and balance
- Strength
- Aerobic stamina

We have already covered flexibility and agility/balance in the previous chapter on biomechanics. This chapter concentrates on strength and aerobic stamina. First, let us summarize why strength and aerobic stamina are so important to the maximizing program.

Strength

Strong muscles stabilize our joints so that they can better absorb shocks. (If you have ever stepped off a low step without realizing that's what you were doing, and therefore didn't tense your muscles, you have felt a jar. This illustrates how important keeping your muscles toned and strong really is.) Developing strong muscles can also improve bone health and thus fight osteoporosis, increase your ability to move freely and perform whatever physical task you reasonably wish, help you control your weight, and as mentioned previously provide you with a reserve capacity in case of illness. Weight lifting, rock climbing, and heavy manual labor improve muscle strength, as does any activity that causes muscles to tire after a few repetitions. The art of strength training lies in doing enough to build your muscles without overstraining them or harming your joints.

Aerobic Stamina

Exercises that improve your physical stamina—your "wind"—and your ability to keep on moving even when you're tired are very important. Not only can they strengthen bones, they also aid in preventing heart disease and stroke and in controlling weight. Brisk walking, running, stair climbing, swimming, bicycling, rowing, cross-country skiing, and other activities that keep your heart rate up for at least twenty consecutive minutes are aerobic exercises. Aerobics, as much as any aspect of exercise, lets you improve the quality of your life. As you become ever more adept, you will find that your overall health and well-being, including your ability to concentrate and the length of time you can work without tiring, all rise. You feel fitter, not just in terms of relieving your arthritis but in every aspect of your life.

Strength and aerobic capacity are necessary for everyone. Obviously, however, they are applicable at different levels for different people. Yet even people whose osteoarthritis is so advanced that they are forced to remain in a wheelchair can exercise to a limited degree to build up their capacity. Gradually the level of exercise they are able to perform increases as their condition improves.

There are two additional advanced aspects to body conditioning: speed and power. Speed requires aerobic capacity and agility, but requires an additional component of its own. It is not needed by everyone, only by people who want to indulge in activities that involve speed, from tennis to sprinting for a bus.

Power is the ability you see in football players, the ability to burst through a defense sometimes against seemingly overwhelming odds. It is a combination of strength and speed, but it has one additional characteristic—the ability to move from an essentially at-rest position to flat-out effort almost instantly. Power training is important for sprinters to teach them how to make a fast start, whereas the race itself depends on speed. Power lets boxers maximize the impact of each punch and gives basketball players that lift that seems to let them defy gravity and hang in the air for an eternity, but aerobic stamina lets them keep doing it. Again, power in this sense is useful but not essential for everyone. If you have osteoarthritis, you will have lost your strength—and your power with it. The first step to regain your power must therefore be to rebuild your strength. Once you have that—and your arthritis under control—your power will return as you train for your sport. Thus, in this chapter, we concentrate on strength and aerobic training, which, along with the flexibility and balance you gain from biomechanics, are the essentials for dealing with your osteoarthritis.

''Use it or lose it'' is the key to all types of fitness. Once you stop exercising, you can quickly lose muscle tone and stamina, become ''tighter,'' and lose much of your agility and balance. Fortunately, the opposite is also true: A little bit of exercise is all it takes to get you started on the road to good physical health. Begin gradually and, as you build your physical and emotional confidence, you'll be able to do more. A moderate but well-designed exercise program is all you need to begin experiencing relief from your joint pain as well as relief from feelings of depression that too often accompany osteoarthritis.

Staying on Track

Most people find that once they are exercising regularly, they not only enjoy it but they hate to stop. They get hooked on exercise—and it's the one addiction that is good for you when not taken to extremes. Nevertheless, at the start, while some people take to exercise like a duck to water, others have to work a little harder to stick with it. If you're in the latter group, here are a few tips to keep you on track.

- Clearly identify your personal exercise goals.
- Celebrate your new program with new clothes/shoes/toys. Rewarding yourself for making this positive change is both desirable and fun.
- Start off gradually, trying not to overdo it.
- If you have the interest and ability, train for competition or an event. There's nothing like the anticipated thrill of victory—or even the pride of finishing—to keep you focused.
- Keep your exercise equipment and gear in plain sight as a reminder.
- Exercise with a partner, if available.
- Work out in the morning. Assuming you sleep well, you may have more energy in the morning. Also, beginning your day with exercise lifts your spirits as well as eases your pain for the rest of the day.
- Combine your work with a workout. For example, enjoy accomplishing work tasks while taking a walk with your coworkers.
- Subscribe to a health magazine and join an exercise club. Reading about and sharing your exercise or activity with others can be very motivating and may bring you new ideas.
- Take it easy when you're not feeling strong. We all have up and down days, and there's no sense letting those down days discourage you. (But do some exercise, even if only a little.)
- If you don't feel like exercising at all one day, do so for at least five minutes. There's a good chance that the five

minutes of exercise will invigorate you and you'll want to continue.
- Keep track of your program and progress with a worksheet like the sample you'll find later in this chapter.
- Have fun!

Some people crave the feelings that come with seeing themselves improve at a task. For them it is very motivating and increases their self-esteem. If you are one of them, please do remember that improvement comes in many forms. You don't have to double the amount of time you spend jogging, or lift twice as much weight, before you can say you've improved. Doing the same workout, but with greater ease, is also a positive sign of your improvement. Just imagine being able to exercise five days a week, when two workouts per week used to tax you beyond endurance. Just a small increase in weight for a difficult lift may represent a tremendous breakthrough. Tracking your improvements can help you celebrate your success.

However, there are many people who feel no great need to keep track of their progress. And as far as we are concerned, there is no need to do so unless it makes you feel good. This is particularly true because progress in any sport or exercise program is not likely to be linear. Even though you show overall improvement, on a day-to-day basis your improvement may fluctuate down and up. If you rely too much on measuring your performance, you are liable to be disappointed and therefore lose motivation. The fact is that if you feel happier and fitter, that is all the progress you need. A well-devised exercise program will achieve those goals.

In this chapter we provide you with the means to create an exercise program that fits all of your personal needs. To do this, we first provide a program of exercises everyone should do to build strength and aerobic stamina. We call this our *basic fitness plan*. Some people, of course, will be unable to handle all the exercises initially because their arthritis simply will not permit it. If this applies to you, do the best you can and you'll soon find yourself able to add activities. Over time, you should be able to handle the entire program.

The second section of this chapter deals with some of the most common arthritis problem areas, such as the back, hips, hands, and knees. We give you exercises that will help you minimize the pain and maximize your mobility in these typical hot-spot areas. All you need to do is identify the areas where you have the most problems, then pick the exercises that correspond to those problem areas and add them to your basic fitness plan. If you have a number of troublesome spots, don't try to solve them all at once. Instead, identify the areas that you feel need the greatest help and concentrate on them first. Over time, as those areas improve, you can move on to others. The combination of your steady overall improvement due to following the basic fitness program, coupled with alleviating your problem areas one or two at a time, will soon have you fitter than you ever thought possible.

The Basic Fitness Plan: Overview

Fortunately, exercise doesn't have to involve a trip to the gym, special clothes and equipment, or more than the amount of special training we provide here. There are plenty of aerobic exercises you can do at home with little or no equipment, wearing any old T-shirt, pair of shorts, or sweat suit you already have. Walking, jogging, dancing, and running—all these can be done at or near home with virtually no equipment. Bicycling is another excellent aerobic exercise, and that old bike you have in the garage will do just fine as long as it's safe to ride. You don't need to buy an expensive new mountain bike. For strength training, which involves giving your muscles resistance, a few weights are all you really need. Joining a gym gives you access to very sophisticated strength-training machines, one for each part of your musculature. Many of these machines can be fun to use, and they let you vary your routine so that you don't get bored. But they are certainly not essential to building up your strength to virtually any level you want to achieve.

Exercise need not be painfully strenuous or take up a great

deal of time in order to be effective. According to the U.S. surgeon general's 1996 report on physical activity and health, "Americans can substantially improve their health and quality of life by including moderate amounts of physical activity in their daily lives . . . physical activity need not be of vigorous intensity for it to improve health." So don't panic! No one is suggesting that you drive yourself into the ground with exercise. Nor do we believe in the axiom, "No pain, no gain." That just isn't so. It is true however, (to quote the same surgeon general's report) that "health benefits appear to be proportional to the amount of activity; thus, every increase in activity adds some benefit." The report goes on to describe what constitutes "moderate" aerobic activity: a brisk thirty-minute walk, forty-five minutes of playing volleyball, thirty minutes of raking leaves or mowing the lawn, or fifteen minutes of running. As you can see, the activity you need to improve your overall health can be a part of your everyday life and need not take excessive time.

Important note: Before embarking on any exercise program, meet with your physician. Your doctor will let you know if there are any reasons why you should restrict your exercise, or will emphasize the importance of performing certain exercises over others. (For example, if you have weak abdominal muscles, your doctor may have you focus on improving them before participating in a general strength-training program, in order to avoid back problems.) Not all physicians are specialists in exercise. Those who are not may refer you to an exercise specialist, such as an exercise physiologist or physical therapist.

Part 1 of the Basic Fitness Plan: *Aerobic Exercise*

Aerobic exercise utilizes your large muscles in a repetitive fashion long enough to get your heart beating at 70 to 85 percent of its maximum rate for at least twenty, but preferably thirty, minutes. Brisk walking, swimming, bicycling, running, aerobic dancing, ice-skating, cross-country skiing, racewalking, jumping rope, rowing, and roller-skating are all aerobic exercises (plus excellent joint lubricators and muscle toners).

Tennis and racquetball can be aerobic if done continuously (without long intermissions between points and games). Vigorous dancing is also an excellent aerobic exercise if done at a rapid pace without stopping.

Naturally, if you are thoroughly out of shape—perhaps having been significantly immobilized by arthritis for a long time—you cannot immediately walk briskly for half an hour. But that is not necessary; all you are seeking to do is to speed up your heart rate for twenty to thirty minutes. If you are very out of shape, that may happen if you walk even quite slowly. So do the best you can. Even if you cannot manage more than a few minutes of activity, don't give up. It may not feel like it at the start, but as you repeat the effort, five minutes will turn to ten, then twenty, then thirty. . . . Your speed will increase, and gradually the pain of your arthritis will wane.

Regular aerobic exercise has been definitely associated with improvement in the symptoms of osteoarthritis. The type of aerobic exercise you choose is unimportant, but you should consider your body's capacity. If you suffer from severe arthritis, have had cartilage removed, or have significant alignment problems in your legs, a high-impact activity that involves running and jumping, such as basketball, football, or soccer, is obviously a bad choice. Instead, if you are suffering from fairly severe osteoarthritis of the weight-bearing joints (low back, hips, knees, ankles, or feet), we recommend that you do only low-impact activities such as water aerobics, swimming, and biking. Those somewhat less affected might become walkers, use a cross-country ski simulator, treadmill, or stair-climbing machine (but if you use such a machine, do your climbing using the technique we described for climbing stairs in the previous chapter on biomechanics). Or you could try elliptical-path training machines, which simulate the motion of jogging without having your feet actually leave the pedals. Equipment technology continuously improves, with more choices becoming available every year. So experiment and find the low- or medium-impact aerobic exercise that works for you.

Remember, no matter what form of exercise you choose, be

sure to drink plenty of water before, after, and during your workout. Even if you don't feel thirsty or don't think you've sweated much, you still have lost fluid during exercise, and that fluid should be replaced. If you become thirsty during exercise, you may already be slightly dehydrated. This impairs your performance and may decrease your motivation—and you won't get as much out of your workout. The best way to replenish your fluids is to drink water (not soda, beer, coffee, or juice). Sports drinks are fine, but they are not necessary and not really helpful unless you're exercising intensely and continuously for an hour or more.

Part 2 of the Basic Fitness Plan: Strength Training

Although we normally associate strength training with bodybuilders and Olympic weight lifters, the truth is that we all benefit from keeping our muscles strong. In addition to increasing muscle mass, strength, and endurance, strength training makes the bones and connective tissues thicker. Thicker connective tissues, in turn, help stabilize our joints. And as part of a well-rounded fitness program, strength training may reduce the risk of heart disease, certain types of cancer, and non-insulin-dependent diabetes.[1] In older adults, or people with advanced arthritis, it reduces the risk of falling by improving balance and decreasing the tendency for a leg to collapse under you due to muscle fatigue.

As fewer and fewer of us are involved in work that is physically taxing enough to give us a good workout, most of us

---

1. A. P. Goldberg, ''Aerobic and Resistive Exercise Modify Risk Factors for Coronary Heart Disease,'' *Med Sci Sports Exerc* 21, no. 6 (1989): 669–74; B. F. Hurley et al., ''Resistive Training Can Reduce Coronary Risk Factors Without Altering VO2 Max or Percent Body Fat,'' *Med Sci Sports Exerc* 20, no. 2 (1988): 150–54; W. J. Miller, W. M. Sherman, and J. L. Ivy, ''Effect of Strength Training on Glucose Tolerance and Post-Glucose Insulin Response,'' *Med Sci Sports Exerc* 16, no. 6 (1984): 539–43; M. A. Smutok et al., ''Aerobic Versus Strength Training for Risk Factor Intervention in Middle-Aged Men at High Risk for Coronary Heart Disease,'' *Metabolism* 42, no. 2 (1993): 177–84; K. H. Koffler et al., ''Strength Training Accelerates Gastrointestinal Transit in Middle-Aged Men and Older Men,'' *Med Sci Sports Exerc* 24, no. 4 (1992): 415–19.

now have to compensate by lifting weights and performing other exercises that stimulate muscle growth. Fortunately, strength-training exercises are very efficient, so that the benefits of a physically active eight-hour workday can be compressed into a brief lifting session.

Rules for Successful Strength Training

Again, as for aerobic exercise, let us suggest some useful ground rules to make your strength-training regimen more efficient and enjoyable.

- *Be sure to breathe!* In most cases, it's best to exhale as you exert yourself, and inhale as you slowly return the weight to the starting position.
- *Focus on good form* rather than on lifting the most weight possible. Don't jerk the weights into position with each lift, then let them crash back down; this uses momentum not muscle. Instead, lift and release slowly. It is not as dramatic, but it's more effective, because you are exercising your muscles throughout the entire exercise, not only half the time. Many trainers believe that you build up your strength as much or more when you gradually lower the weights as when you gradually raise them. It's always harder to complete any exercise when you're doing it slowly because your muscles are worked through a range of motion without the help of momentum. It's also safer to perform these exercises slowly, reducing the risk of further injury through improper technique.
- *Never lift more than you can handle.* Trying to do one or two "super lifts" with a very heavy weight is not a good idea and is completely unnecessary for you to progress.
- *Use of constant muscle contraction during a lift.* Constant muscle tension means that you flex (tighten) the muscle you are working throughout the entire range of motion of a particular exercise, essentially maintaining the tension on the muscle. This has the effect of recruiting more muscle fibers to do the work. The reason bodybuilders and others (including you!) should use this principle is because it teaches you

how to use your muscles more efficiently, thus improving your biomechanics.

To give you an example of how this works, reach up with your right hand and touch your nose with your fingers. Now do it again, this time concentrating on flexing your bicep muscle throughout the entire range as you slowly reach for your nose. You will see that, in the first case, your body did almost no work. Whereas in the second, the muscles in your arm got a meaningful workout. If you repeat the second approach ten times, your arm will be noticeably tired. If you do it daily, your arm will become noticeably stronger.

- *Your ideal routine should cover all major muscle groups,* specifically:

> calves and thighs
> hips and buttocks
> back, chest, and shoulders
> arms and hands
> abdominals

You don't have to do these areas all on the same day. Just try to cover all of them twice a week, always starting with the larger muscles first.

Exercise experts say that it's best to allow a day of rest between workouts for any particular body part. (And of course you should not exercise an area that is still sore from a prior workout. That's neither comfortable, wise, nor necessary.) Some people perform all of the upper body exercises on one day and work on the lower body the next. (the "upper-lower" strength workout). Others do the whole routine every other day. Many enjoy separating their exercises into those that push weight away from the body and those that pull weight towards the body (the "push-pull" strength workout). Do whichever feels best to you.

- *Don't overdo it.* Don't try to do fifty different exercises a day. Instead, begin with a routine that includes a few exercises, as many as you can manage easily. Then add new ones as you gain strength and confidence. It's likely that you'll want to continue to add new exercises when you see and feel the benefits you're getting. But take it slowly; add only one new exercise at a time, and be sure not to over-emphasize any one muscle group.

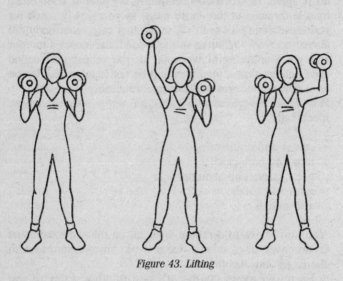

Figure 43. Lifting

For some, lifting causes pain or discomfort if the weight is moved through the entire range of motion. Rather than trying to work through this pain, or simply skipping this exercise, try moving the weight through a limited range. For example, suppose you are doing a shoulder pass using dumbbells. Instead of pushing the dumbbells all the way above your head until you gently lock your elbows, push them only halfway up before returning to the starting position. You will still experience significant benefit from the lift, and gradually you'll be able to push farther. This partway approach will open more lifting options for you as you progress.

• *If you feel pain or "funny" feelings in your joints while exercising, stop.* You may be doing the exercise improperly, you may be using too much weight, or perhaps you should try to build those same muscles using a different exercise. (A useful tip is to ask someone who's experienced with strength training whether you're doing your new lift correctly. If you're at a gym, there are usually experienced lifters or professional trainers around who'll be glad to share their knowledge with you for a few minutes.) If the problem persists—particularly if changing exercises and weights doesn't help—consult your doctor or physical therapist about the problem.

- *If you feel dizzy, faint, or light-headed, or are panting for breath, you are overdoing things.* Take it easier. If the problem persists, see your physician.
- *Pace yourself as you go through your routine.* Do your bench presses, for example, then rest briefly until your breath has almost returned to normal before moving on to the next activity. But don't sit down to rest. Walk around, so that you don't cool down too much. If you find that you must wait several minutes between exercises, you're pushing yourself too hard. You may need to work on your aerobic exercises to increase your wind and lift lighter weights until your muscles get used to the demands you're placing on them.
- *Don't rush through your routine just because you can.* Work at a moderate pace, taking short breaks between sets and between exercises. If your routine is too easy, use heavier weights and do more repetitions, or add new exercises.
- *Forget that slogan, "No pain, no gain."* While you should probably feel some muscle soreness the day after you exercise, especially at the beginning or after you advance to a new stage in your development, if your muscles are constantly sore, you're overdoing it.
- *Devise a routine that you can, and will, stick with.* But of course, having a routine doesn't mean you should never vary it. That's boring! There are more than two hundred different types of strength training exercises. So every few sessions, replace some old exercises with new ones. This will help keep your program interesting and provide your body with a continuous source of new challenges.

• *Use a spotter when using free weights,* if possible. The spotter will be there to prevent injury should you lose control and can help you with difficult final lifts if needed. Of course, if you're working out at home and no spotter is available, you won't be able to follow this advice. Don't make that an excuse for not working out! Dumbbells can be used safely without a spotter. If you are unable to control them, let them fall harmlessly to your sides. However, when you use barbells that cross your chest, you *must* control them. *So if no spotter is available, use lighter weights!*

The Basic Fitness Plan

Aerobics

The basic aerobic plan is extremely easy to describe: Simply do any aerobic exercise for at least twenty minutes or until you feel thoroughly warm and you are slightly short of breath. This means that you are able to speak fairly easily but do not have enough breath to carry on an extended conversation. You should not be panting and gasping. On the other hand, you should not be able to conduct a business meeting comfortably either!

The specific aerobic exercise you choose can be any one you enjoy. You can vary it each time you work out, or combine two or more in a cross-training session. For example, bicycle a few miles to a park, lock up the bike and walk briskly for a mile, then end with the return ride home. This sort of mixed exercise has several advantages over either walking or bicycling exclusively. For most people, it's more fun; it uses different muscles; you can push yourself a little harder during three short segments than for a longer single one; and it reduces the risk of a repetition-caused irritation to specific joints. This benefit is especially significant for people with osteoarthritis, and we strongly encourage cross training within individual aerobic exercise sessions or by alternating modes of exercise during the week.

How hard should you exercise? For ordinary fitness training, your *goal* should be to keep your heart rate up for no less than thirty minutes, without excessive shortness of breath. Of course, it may take you some time to reach that goal if you are now out of training. But many good things are worth striving for—and relieving your arthritis is surely one of them.

If you also want to develop speed, you need to spend about a third of the time you are doing your aerobic exercise doing it fast. Running, cycling, or swimming sprints should be interspersed with normal aerobic activity. At the end of each sprint, you should be out of breath but not gasping. Your breathing should return to its normal level.

No individual exercises are better for you than any other provided they give you a sufficient workout. However, you should do exercises which do not aggravate any arthritis problem areas from which you may be suffering. Rather, you should "work around" those specifically vulnerable places by doing other exercises. The chart on the next page has some examples.

There are eight basic parts of the body that need strengthening two to three times per week. As mentioned, some people do exercises for each part of the body in a single workout session. However, if this proves too much for you, you can alternate between body parts as long as you work each muscle group at least two times each week. Fewer workouts do not allow significant improvements to be made. On the other hand, you should generally not exercise any body part more than every other day. Although your body enjoys consistent movement and toning, it also needs appropriate recuperation time between exercise.

When choosing which part of your body to exercise, you may want to exert more effort to strengthen areas that you feel are weak or that are giving you trouble. Remember, though, not to spend so much time on any one body part that you ignore the others, and always remember to work the larger muscle groups first. For example, work your chest muscles before your arm muscles.

REPS AND SETS

How many times you do a particular exercise depends on your goals. Weight-lifting regimens are broken down into sets, with each set consisting of a number of repetitions, or reps. For example, three sets of ten reps each means you lift the weight ten times, take a 15–30 second break, lift it ten more times, take a brief break, and lift it a final ten times. You take a break between sets because the last couple of reps in each set should be tiring and somewhat difficult to do. Therefore, you need a moment for your muscles to recover. Sixty seconds should be ample.

Generally speaking, two to three sets per exercise is a good goal. In order to warm up the muscles and joints to avoid injury, we recommend that you use a lighter weight and do more reps in your first set, then increase the weight and do fewer reps in the second and third sets.

The number of reps you do per set depends on what you're trying to achieve. Here's the rule of thumb: More reps at lower weight yields more endurance and tone than strength. For example, if you are a woman with strong, muscular thighs, you may not want to build them any further. Thus, to maintain their strength and endurance but not increase their size, you would choose more reps (say, twenty to twenty-five) at a lower weight until your muscle(s) fatigue (that is, until you can't do any more reps). Fewer reps at higher weight produce more strength but less endurance. So if you want stronger arms—perhaps to help you with a hobby you enjoy such as home improvement—you will want to use heavier weights. Most people working on enhancing general health and fitness do eight to twelve reps per set until fatigue, since that is a good compromise between building endurance and building muscle.

People who wish to build up their power use weights that are on the heavy side, with fewer reps per set (one to five). They also do each exercise with more "explosive" (i.e., sudden exertion) force. And, of course, they exercise more frequently—at least five times per week in most cases—to build true power. Power lifting has a much higher risk for injury

AEROBICS

		RUN/JOG	WALKING	BICYCLING/ STATIONARY	SWIMMING	CROSS-COUNTRY SKI MACHINE	STAIR CLIMBER	GLIDER	ROWING
		RECOMMENDED AEROBIC EXERCISES THAT MINIMIZE STRESS ON PAINFUL JOINT AREAS							
Painful Joint Areas	Ankle			x	x			x	x
	Knee			x	x	x	x	x	x
	Hip			x	x			x	
	Low Back			x	x			x	
	Shoulder	x	x		x		x		
	Neck		x		x	x	x		x
	Hand/Elbow	x	x		x				

due to the increase in lifting intensity that is required to achieve results. So we don't recommend this as a goal for OA sufferers.

How many pounds should you lift? The trick is to choose a weight that fatigues your muscles so that you can only just manage the last couple of reps in each set. It doesn't matter if it's one pound or one hundred—select the weight that's right for you. If you are unable to perform more than seven reps with the weight you have chosen, you are using too much weight. Conversely, if you can do more than twelve reps without much difficulty, you probably need to add some weight.

When you find the right weight, make sure that you are able to hold your form on those last two difficult reps. If your last rep is so tough that you cannot move back to the starting position slowly and under control but have to virtually drop the weights, then you are using too much weight.

So do push yourself to a sensible limit—but don't overdo it. Don't try to lift more than you can comfortably (while taxing your muscles at the appropriate, limited times). You're not training for the Olympics, no one's keeping score, you don't have to worry about impressing anyone. Your only goal is to get stronger, safely.

The Core Program

The following exercises form the core of your basic fitness program. These are the exercises that should be done by everyone at least twice a week. The degree of difficulty depends mostly on how much weight you choose. However, in some cases, we show you other tricks to increase difficulty. Obviously, the level you choose depends on how fit you are. As you become fitter, your level of difficulty will inch upward. You will hardly notice the improvement at first, but after a few months you will be surprised at the progress you've made.

One final word about weight training. It can be done low-tech with barbells and dumbbells, or high-tech with computerized machines at the gym. You can even take the no-tech approach, lifting heavy cans of soup (one pound) or bricks (four pounds). Whether you work out at home with barbells and laundry bottles or at the gym surrounded by hundreds of thousands of dollars worth of equipment is up to you. People argue that one approach is better than another, adamantly insisting that free weights are better than machines or vice versa. Which is better? There is no reliable research on the subject, so our answer is whichever one works for you. Try the free weights, weight machines, and computerized devices at your gym, if you belong. Pick the approach you like and with which you will most readily stick. By the way, there's nothing wrong with combining free weights, weight machines, and computerized weight machines. For many people, such a varied strength-training program is more fun.

We show you these exercises using free weights. However, you'll have no trouble transferring them to weight machines or computerized machines if that is your preference. So for now, you only need a few pieces of equipment:

- a sturdy bench, preferably padded
- two adjustable-weight dumbbells, or a set of dumbbells of varying weights
- ankle weights (one to five lbs.)
- a towel or mat
- a barbell to which you can attach various weights (optional)

There are only nine parts of your body that need strength training. One requires three separate exercises, one requires two exercises, and the rest require only one exercise each. Thus the basic program calls for twelve exercises. We call them the magic dozen. The nine areas are:

- Shoulders
- Arms (biceps and triceps, the front and back of your arms)
- Chest
- Upper back
- Lower back
- Abdominals
- Buttocks (usually referred to as ''gluts''—pronounced ''gloots''—short for gluteus maximus)

- Thighs (front of thigh or quadriceps, that part of your thighs that forms your lap; hamstrings, the back of your thighs; and inner thighs)
- Calves

The Magic Dozen

Our tendency when we exert ourselves is to hold our breath. This just makes the work harder. Our bodies need oxygen to function properly and to prevent blood pressure from dangerously going up. Get into the habit of breathing when you exercise. Inhale on *every* exertion; exhale on *every* release. If you can't remember to breathe, count aloud each rep. Saying ''one,'' pause, ''two,'' pause, ''three,'' pause . . . forces you to breathe.

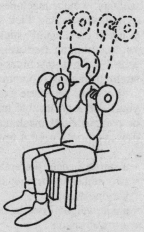

Figure 44. Shoulder Press

SHOULDERS

SHOULDER PRESS
Sitting with your feet flat on the floor and your back straight, hold the dumbbells with an overhand grip and raise them to shoulder level.

Holding your chest up, your back straight, and your elbows in, press the dumbbells straight up toward the ceiling. Slowly lower the weights to the starting position and repeat eight to twelve times. The degree of difficulty for this exercise depends on the amount of weight you are lifting. So vary it accordingly. You can also do this while standing, which adds slightly to the difficulty.

ARMS: BICEPS

BICEPS CURL

Standing with your feet about shoulder-width apart, hold a barbell or two free weights with your arms hanging in front of you and your hands a little less than shoulder-width apart, palms facing away from you. Your elbows should press gently against your sides.

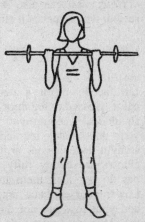

Keeping your elbows against your sides, raise the bar up to your chest, until it just about touches. Then gradually lower it back to the starting position.

Figure 45. Biceps Curl

Note: Be sure to keep your elbows in place and not to swing them forward or back. Also keep your body upright and still; don't swing back and forth as you lift and release. You can work slightly different "angles" of the biceps by using a wider or narrower grip.

The degree of difficulty here depends on the weight. If you are using too much weight, you will find yourself moving your elbows or arching your back to get some momentum. If so, use a lighter weight.

ARMS: TRICEPS

TRICEPS EXTENSION

Standing with your feet shoulder-width apart, hold a dumbbell with both hands above and slightly behind your head. Wrap your hands around the dumbbell's handle with your palms facing up, supporting the upper weight plates.

Lower the dumbbell behind your head until your forearms are at least parallel with the floor, pause for a second or so, then lift the weight back up to the beginning position. Adjust the weight to suit your ability. Repeat eight to twelve times.

Note: You can also do this while seated, which makes it slightly easier.

CHEST

PUSH-UP
Lie facedown on a mat or towel, palms pressed to the floor next to your shoulders. Keeping your body stiff, your abdominals in, and your back straight, extend your arms until your elbows are nearly fully straightened but do not lock them into position. Lower yourself back until your face and your hips are not quite touching the floor and repeat. If you cannot complete eight to twelve full push-ups, do the exercise resting on your knees instead of your toes. If you are more advanced, increase the number

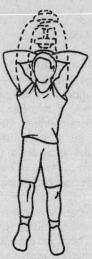

Figure 46. Triceps Extension

of push-ups to twenty, and then make them more difficult by doing them *very slowly*.

Note: The bad news is that push-ups are difficult, especially if you have never exercised a day in your life and if you are lugging around some extra pounds (after all, you are pushing up all your body weight). The good news is that this is an exercise where you see improvement quickly. If the first day you can do only one push-up, that's fine. Your next workout you'll be able to do two. In two weeks you'll be doing ten—and feeling smug.

UPPER BACK

BENCH ROW
Place your left hand and your left knee on a bench, leaving your right foot on the ground and your right hand free. Keep your trunk and your shoulders parallel to the floor. You should now be in a semikneeling position. Now pick up a dumbbell

with your right hand and let the weight hang directly under your right shoulder. With your palm facing in (toward the bench), lift your elbow straight up toward the ceiling, much as if you were trying to start a lawn mower, but without the jerk. Keep the dumbbell close to your body and keep your trunk as stable as possible. Slowly lower the dumbbell back to the starting position. Repeat eight to twelve times, then repeat the exercise with your left hand.

The degree of difficulty here is again based on how much weight you are lifting. Choose accordingly.

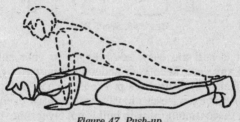

Figure 47. Push-up

LOWER BACK

BACKWARD SIT-UP

Lie facedown on a towel or mat, with your arms pillowing your head. Lift your head and chest, at the same time as your feet and legs, a couple of inches off of the ground (you shouldn't be able to lift very far). As you lift your upper body, look at the floor so you don't extend your head and neck too far back. Keep your legs straight. Your back will be slightly arched and you should feel the lower back muscles working. Hold this position for a couple of seconds, then slowly come back to the starting position. Repeat until your lower back muscles are fatigued.

If you do more than twenty reps of this exercise, make it more difficult by extending your arms straight out in front of

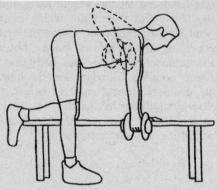

Figure 48. Bench Row

you. If it is still too easy, add weights to your ankles and wrists. In any case, keep your abdominal muscles tight.

Individuals with acute back problems such as disk problems should do this exercise cautiously, and perhaps even one leg at a time, discontinuing if pain builds up. Over time, however, you should find that this exercise considerably reduces your back pain.

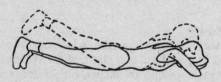

Figure 49. Backward Sit-up

ABDOMINALS

ABDOMINAL CRUNCH

Lie flat on your back with your knees bent. Push your heels slightly into the floor so that your lower back is flat. Cross your hands in front of you and lay them on your chest. And—need we say it?—hold in those abs.

Slowly curl your upper body up and forward as far as is comfortable for you. Slowly return to the starting position. (Some people can get higher than others. This is not a competition. As long as your abs are tightened, even if you can raise yourself only a couple of inches you are working.) Challenge yourself; start out with twenty reps and increase to fifty. When they become easy, try these variations:

- Perform the same exercise with your hands behind your head (Figure 50).
- Perform the same exercise but twist to the left or right as you come up, thus working the sides of your abdominals. You should use your arms to cradle your head when performing this variation.
- Keep your feet a few inches off the ground while you crunch (this is harder than it sounds!). Do not do this if you feel pain in your back.
- Hook your feet under something heavy and "crunch" up slightly farther than you normally can.

Note: With abdominal crunches, it is especially important to breathe—out on the way up, in on the way down. Also, form is crucial here. Find a spot on the ceiling and focus on it. As you crunch, your back, neck, and head stay in a straight line—it's your abdominal muscles pulling you up, rather than your neck doing all the work. Finally, your hands are only supporting your head; don't use your hands to push your head and body up. And watch out for your elbows. They should be out to the side, not forward. They have a natural tendency to creep forward, especially as your abs get tired. If you can see your elbows out of the corners of your eyes, they are too far forward. Pull 'em back.

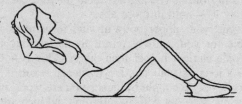

Figure 50. Advanced Abdominal Crunch

BUTTOCKS

SQUAT

Stand with your feet about shoulder-width apart, one to two feet in front of a weight bench (positioned so that when you squat down, your buttocks would sit squarely on the bench). Extend your arms at shoulder height, parallel to the floor, or cross your arms and keep them in front of you at shoulder height.

Keeping your head and chest up and your back straight, squat down until your buttocks are just barely above the bench. Hold there for a moment, then stand up. Your knees should be straightly aligned over your feet as you squat. Repeat eight to twelve times. This exercise has the advantage of also helping your thighs, which is especially good because, being very large and powerful muscles, they need extra work to make them strong.

You can make this exercise easier by holding something stable like a railing or doorknob as you squat. And you can make it gradually harder by using an increasingly heavy barbell (held behind the head on the shoulders) as you perform the exercise.

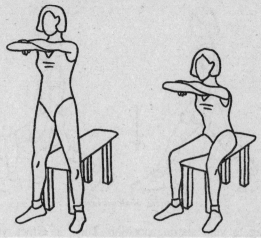

Figure 51. Squat

THIGHS: QUADRICEPS AND HAMSTRINGS

MODIFIED LUNGE

Stand with your feet about a foot apart, holding a dumbbell in each hand. Then move one foot one large step (one or two feet, depending on how long your legs are) forward.

Keeping your back straight and head up, try to bend the front leg until your thigh is parallel to the ground. Then push back with the front leg (push the heel into the floor) to return to the starting position. The predominant movement should be more up and down than forward and back. You should feel the thigh muscles in the front leg working with this exercise. Do eight to twelve repetitions on one side, then switch and do the same procedure on the other side.

You can make this exercise easier or more difficult by changing the amount of weight you carry. You can also make it harder by converting it to a full "walking" lunge. You do this by moving forward after you have lunged, rather than

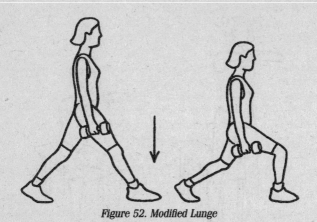

Figure 52. Modified Lunge

returning to your starting position. Thus, in effect, you are taking large forward strides with a deep lunge between each step. If you have hip or knee arthritis, the modified lunge is preferred over the walking lunge.

THIGHS: INNER

To strengthen your inner thigh, lie on your right side, cradling your head with your right hand. Cross your leg over your right thigh, planting your left foot down flat in front of you. Lean slightly forward, using your left hand to support you.

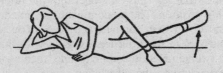

Figure 53. Inner Thigh

Keeping your knee straight, lift your right leg about ten inches off the floor, while concentrating on contracting the muscles in your thigh. Hold the position for five seconds, then lower the leg. Repeat eight to twelve times, then turn onto your left side and do the same with your left leg. Add resistance with light ankle weights (no more than five pounds) if you can easily do twenty repetitions without fatigue.

Note: If you belong to a gym that has a hip adduction machine, we strongly recommend that you learn the proper way to use it. Used correctly, this is a terrific machine also for working the area.

THIGHS: OUTER

To strengthen your outer thigh, lie on your right side, your right arm under your head. Keeping your knee straight, lift your left leg about ten inches off the ground, hold the position for three to five seconds, then lower it so that it nearly touches the floor about one foot in front of you, or lower it so that it gently glances the resting leg. Concentrate on contracting the muscles in your thigh as you perform this movement. Repeat eight to twelve times, then turn onto your left side and do the same with your right leg. Add resistance with light ankle weights (no more than five pounds) if you can easily do twenty repetitions without fatigue. Again, if your gym has special equipment, such as a hip abductor, designed to work this muscle area, seek assistance from a professional trainer to learn how to use it properly.

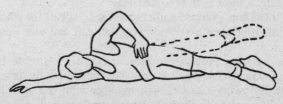

Figure 54. Outer Thigh

CALVES

CALF RAISE

Stand with your feet slightly less than hip width apart. Raise up onto the balls of both feet (your tiptoes), with your weight evenly distributed over them. Hold the position for three to five seconds, then gently lower to your starting position. Repeat twelve to fifteen times, or until you feel a ''burn'' in your calves.

If you become adept at this basic exercise, try this more advanced variation. Stand on a stair, board, or platform raised a few inches off the ground. The raised step should be next to a wall, desk, or rail you can

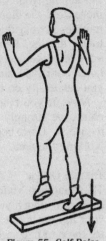

Figure 55. Calf Raise

hold to keep your balance. Place your right foot near the edge of the step so that the ball of your foot is on the edge and your heel is hanging off. Your left foot should be off the ground.

Holding on to the wall or other support, drop your right heel, then raise it. Keep your toes firmly in place, your body straight, and your right knee straight but not locked. Move only up and down, not back and forth, and do not sway or bounce. Repeat twelve times or until you feel a ''burn'' in your calf. Repeat with the other leg.

To make this exercise harder, carry a dumbbell (in your left hand when you are exercising your left calf and vice versa).

So far we have presented a basic exercise program to build your aerobic and strength fitness. We summarize the program on the following chart. Taken together with the stretching, flexibility, and agility/balance exercises described in the previous chapter, you now have a basic fitness program that will keep you healthy. Moreover, it can be adapted to nearly every level of fitness so that however weak you may be at the beginning, you can get started. And once you start, you *will* improve. Gradually you will become more limber, more resilient and tireless, and stronger. As you do, your arthritis will start to improve. Since you will be taking the supplements at the same time, that improvement will be helped by the regeneration of some of your cartilage. Before too long, you will be feeling much better.

Exercising the "Hot Spots"

Though most people can handle the basic exercise program, not everyone is at the same level in terms of physical ability, especially if you factor in the various aspects of fitness: aerobics, strength, flexibility, and agility/balance. Unfortunately, some people are so immobilized by osteoarthritis that almost no "exercise" is possible. In the worst cases, muscular stimulation by the application of electricity, or having a therapist help move the patient's limbs, is just about the only activity the body is capable of doing.

Some people are slightly better off and may be able to do *isometric exercise.* Isometric exercise is a method of contracting the muscles without moving the joints. Isometric exercise can allow you to maintain some muscle tone without aggravating an inflamed joint.

If you are in the challenging position of falling into either of these categories, you should be under the supervision of a professional exercise therapist. All we can add is that you *can* be helped. Don't give up. Do whatever exercise you can, and you may reach the point where our biomechanical, aerobic, and "magic dozen" strength exercises are no longer beyond you.

For those of you who are luckier because your condition has not progressed as far, arthritis can still be a stubborn problem. Therefore, there is one more step you need to take to maximize the arthritis cure: You must add some aerobic and strength-training exercises to your workout each day to help

THE MAGIC DOZEN PROGRESS CHART

	EXERCISES		MON.	TUES.	WED.	THURS.	FRI.	SAT.	SUN.
	Shoulders	Shoulder Press							
	Arms	Biceps Curl							
		Triceps Extension							
	Chest	Push-Ups							
Core Program (2–4 times per week)	Upper Back	Bench Rows							
	Lower Back	Backward Sit-Up							
	Abdominals	Abdominal Crunch							
	Buttocks	Squat							
	Thighs	Modified Lunge							
		Inner Thigh							
		Outer Thigh							
	Calves	Calf Raise							

Check the box when you do the exercise.

protect the joints that are especially problematic for you. You must do this for two reasons: to strengthen muscles that can take some of the load off your most painful joints, and to protect the joints from being reinjured over time and redeveloping the osteoarthritis you are in the process of curing!

In some cases, doing these extra exercises may seem easier said than done. You should logically be spending more of your exercise time on the areas that are the most problematic for you, and it may be hard to get yourself motivated to do this. In general, people tend to enjoy the things they can do easily and dislike those they find hard. We know of no easy answer to this, but we can make you a proposition: Try doing the "difficult" exercises for just four weeks. Most probably you will be surprised by three things: how much better the "difficult" area feels; how much better the other areas of your body feel (remember, everything is interconnected); and, most surprising, how much more you enjoy actually doing the exercises. It's a safe bet that if you do your auxiliary exercises on top of your basic fitness plan for four weeks, you won't want to quit.

Well over half of all cases of disability caused by osteoarthritis are due to the disease striking in the knees or hips. Consequently, we first describe special exercises for these areas. Then we move on to the other main problem areas for osteoarthritis: hands and fingers; back; shoulders, elbows, and wrists; ankles and feet.

As with the basic fitness plan, you can do this auxiliary program with a lot of equipment or very little. We provide you with exercises that require the minimum possible. You'll need:

- a set of rubber tubing or resistance bands with handles and a waist belt (available at athletic stores, physical therapists' offices, and surgical supply outlets for about $20 to $40)
- a rubber band
- a set of one- to two-pound ankle weights
- a "squeeze" ball (or set of squeeze balls of varying degrees of resistance). These can be purchased at health product

stores or surgical supply houses, or ask your physical therapist where you can buy one. Look for one that maintains constant resistance as you squeeze it through the entire range of motion.

Let's get started with strengthening those problem spots. Here are the exercises:

Knees

The most important thing you can do for your knees is to strengthen the muscles all around them without placing excess pressure on the knee joints themselves. To this end, the first thing you can do is to choose aerobic exercises that strengthen your legs as well as serve their main function of building your stamina. Obviously, the best exercises for this are those that *move* your knees but don't expose them to too much pressure or jarring. Bicycling is probably the best all-around exercise for this. However, in the gym, you may also find stationary ski machines and "running" machines where your feet never leave the ground or "jar" down between steps.

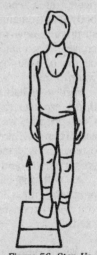

In addition to these aerobic workout suggestions, here are some simple strength-building ideas for the muscles around your knees.

STEP UP

One of the very best ways to strengthen your quadriceps, hamstrings, and buttocks (which will help

Figure 56. Step Up

you with hip problems) is one of the simplest exercises of all. All you do is step up onto a stair (or large book, wooden block, etc.), pulling yourself all the way up until you are standing on the stop and your working leg is straightened. Don't "push off," but consciously contract your thigh muscles as you step up. Move up slowly to avoid momentum aiding the exercise, then *slowly* step back down. Do up to thirty reps, then repeat with the other leg. If the exercise becomes too easy, use a taller step. If the exercise is too hard at the start, give yourself a boost by hanging onto a railing, chair back, or door knob.

WALL SLIDE

Another valuable exercise to help your legs without harming your knees is to stand with your back to a wall, feet about shoulder-width apart. The back of your feet should be ten to eighteen inches away from the wall.

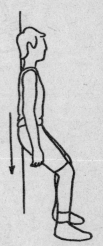

Slide your back down the wall until your knees are bent at no more than a 90-degree angle (the angle you are most comfortable with at first may only be a 45-degree one. Don't fret, you will gradually improve). Hold position for five to twenty seconds, slide back up. Repeat five to fifteen times.

Note: This exercise is surprisingly challenging. Do not despair if at first you can do only five reps for five sec-

Figure 57. Wall Slide

onds each. Also, you need some traction so your feet don't slide forward. Either work on carpet (*not* a throw rug) or wear sneakers.

These two exercises, practiced regularly, will strengthen your thighs sufficiently. And you can augment them by walking a lot, especially up steep hills. In addition, if you have access to a health club or gym, chances are you'll have access to both a leg press and a hamstring-curl machine. These are among the most important machines for strengthening your buttocks, hips, and thighs. They do not do anything you cannot do at home, but they get the strengthening job done faster, and they are fun to use. If you are really having problems with your legs, being able to use these machines is almost reason enough for joining a gym. Of course, the personnel at your gym will show you how to use them. . . . It's very simple.

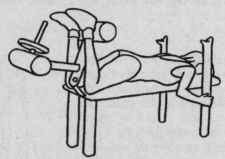

Figure 58. Hamstring Curl Machine

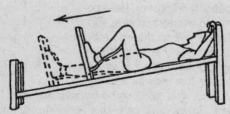

Figure 59. Leg Press Machine

MODIFIED LEG SQUAT

This exercise requires the rubber tubing device mentioned earlier. Attach one end of the tube to a heavy or fixed object that will not give (such as the leg of a heavy sofa).

Begin by bending down a few inches and stepping on the rubber tubing so that, when you stand up straight, the tubing is taut. Stand with your feet about shoulder-width apart, placing your right foot on the tube, and holding the handle in your right arm. Then, lift your left foot off the ground so that you are balancing on one foot. Hold onto a rail or chair for balance if you wish. Keeping your back straight and your head up, bend your right knee to about a 45-degree angle. Hold for five seconds and come back up to the starting position. Do eight to twelve reps. Vary the length of the tubing to add or lessen the amount of resistance. Repeat on the left side.

If the one-handed pull is too difficult, do the two-handed pull instead. This is the same exercise, except that you stand on the tubing with both feet and hold the handles or ends in both hands. Remember to keep your elbows straight. Then proceed as above.

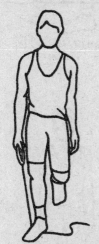

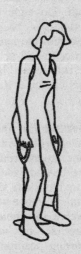

Figure 60A. Modified Leg Squat   *Figure 60B. Modified Leg Squat*

A selection of these exercises, repeated every two or three days as an addition to your basic workout, will greatly strengthen your legs and help protect your knees. As a bonus, you will also have helped protect your hip joints. Here are some further exercises, however, that you can do to strengthen this vital area.

Hips

RESISTED HIP FLEXION

Stand with one end of the tubing attached to your right ankle and the other to a sofa leg. Shift all your weight to your left foot. Keeping your knee straight but not locked, raise your right leg slightly and smoothly move it forward about twelve to eighteen inches. Hold for three seconds and come back to the starting position. Do eight to twelve reps. Step forward or backward to increase or decrease the tension on the tubing in order to add or lessen the amount of resistance, and hence the difficulty, of this exercise. Repeat on the opposite side.

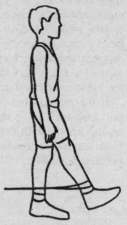

Figure 61. Resisted Hip Flexion

RESISTED HIP ABDUCTION

Stand with your feet together with the tube around your left ankle and passing behind your right ankle, and secured to a sofa leg. Keeping your knee straight, move your leg outward about twelve to eighteen inches. Hold for three seconds and come back to the starting position. Do eight to twelve reps. As before, step toward or away from the "anchored" base of the tubing to add to or lessen the amount of resistance. Then repeat with the other leg.

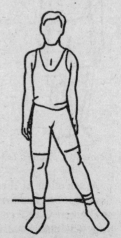

Figure 62. Resisted Hip Abduction

RESISTED HIP ADDUCTION

This is the exact opposite of the prior exercise. Stand with your feet together with the tubing around your right ankle and anchored to a sofa leg. Then pull your right leg across your body to the left, as far as you comfortably can. Repeat eight to twelve times, then turn around so that your left side is facing the anchor and loop your left ankle through the other end. Repeat the exercise with the left leg the same as you did with the right.

When you try them, you'll find that not only are these additional exercises easy to do but, after a few weeks, you'll also find that they are helping you considerably in keeping your arthritis at bay.

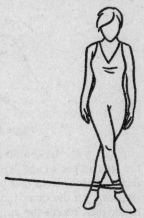

Figure 63. Resisted Hip Adduction

Hands and Fingers

Everyone who has suffered from arthritis in the joints of their hands and fingers knows how miserable this condition can be. You can help the situation by exercise. And for those people who don't especially enjoy exercise, there is an added bonus: These range of motion exercises are very easy to do, they do not make you pant, and you don't need to shower afterward!

FULL, HALF, AND TOP FINGER BENDS

With the thumb and first finger of your right hand, bend the first finger of the left hand at the bottom joint (knuckle) until you feel a stretch. Hold position for five seconds, then release. Repeat with the thumb and other three fingers on the left hand, then reverse positions and sequentially bend all four fingers and the thumb on the right hand.

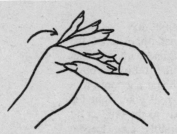

Figure 64. Full Finger Bend

Next, with the thumb and first finger of right hand, bend the first finger of the left hand at the middle joint until you feel a stretch. Hold that position for five seconds and release. Repeat with the other three fingers and the thumb on the left hand, then repeat the exercises on all five digits on the right hand.

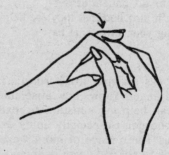

Figure 65. Half Finger Bend

Finally, with the thumb and first finger of the right hand, bend the first finger of the left hand at the last (''top'') joint until you feel a stretch. Hold position for five seconds and release. Repeat with the other three fingers and the thumb on the left hand, then repeat the exercise on the right hand.

You will probably be astonished by how much more easily you can grip things after you have assiduously done these finger exercises for a few weeks.

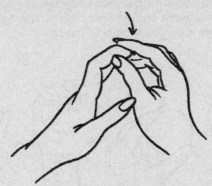

Figure 66. Top Finger Bend

SQUEEZE BALL EXERCISES

Here are four exercises with a squeeze ball to strengthen your hands while increasing coordination. Remember that the force on joints (including the finger joints) increases when the muscle tone drops. Maintaining strength in the fingers and hands is an important way to fight osteoarthritis in these areas. Do these exercises, with both hands, at least two to three times per week. You can do them at home in the morning while reading the paper, during short breaks at work, in the evening, while walking, while watching television or talking on the phone. Perform multiple repetitions until you feel the muscles fatigue.

The exercises should be done in a group, one after the other, and then repeated. Do each exercise by holding the squeeze for a count of three seconds, performing ten reps of each. They are:

- Squeeze the ball with your entire hand.
- Squeeze with your thumb and each individual finger, in turn. (Figure 67 shows only the thumb and the index finger, but be sure to exercise each of the other three fingers as well.)

- Squeeze the ball with just your fingertips.
- Squeeze it between each of your fingers, making sure to do this between each finger on both hands.

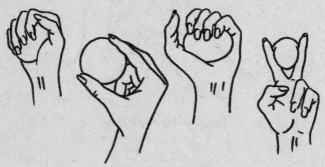

Figure 67. Squeeze Ball

FINGER EXTENSION

Place a rubber band on the outside of the fingers and the thumb. Now try to separate your fingers while using your thumb as an "anchor." This should cause your finger muscles to fatigue after a few repetitions. If it doesn't, use a stronger rubber band.

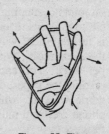

Figure 68. Finger Extension

AGILE FINGER STRETCH

Finally, two additional squeeze ball exercises that make your fingers stronger and more agile:

- Move two balls in your hand in a continuous circling of each other. Do this exercise for fifteen to thirty seconds. Repeat for at least three sets.

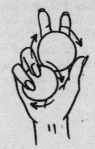

Figure 69. Squeeze Ball

• Thread the ball through your fingers. Do this exercise for fifteen to thirty seconds. Again, do at least three sets.

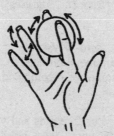

Figure 70. Squeeze Ball

The Back

The next most problematic area for many people is the back. The following exercise is terrific for loosening and strengthening the entire back. If this is a problem area for you, be sure to add this exercise to your basic program.

"SWIMMING"

Lie flat on the floor, facedown, a pillow under your stomach (optional), your face resting on a small pillow or rolled-up towel. Stretch both arms forward, as you would if you were swimming the crawl. Then, lift your left leg and right arm off the ground at the same time. Hold them out straight, about four to six inches off the floor for five seconds. Gently lower them to the ground, then do the same with the right leg and left arm. Repeat on both sides five to ten times.

You can make this exercise harder by placing light weights around your wrists and ankles.

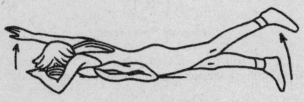

Figure 71. "Swimming"

Shoulders, Elbows, and Wrists

To help protect these joints, you need to do arm-strengthening exercises. Here are some we recommend.

UPRIGHT ROW

This exercise works your forearms and your shoulders. Stand with your feet shoulder-width apart, holding a barbell (or hand weights). With your elbows pointing outward, pull the bar toward your chin. Stop when the weight is just below your chin. At that point, the tips of your elbows should be at about ear level and should be pointed outward, like fully spread wings. Now lower the weight to the starting position. Your elbows should be higher than your hands throughout this lift. Repeat eight to twelve times, selecting the appropriate weight to make the exercise harder or easier, as needed.

Note: You can work slightly different areas of the same muscles by doing this exercise with a wider or narrower grip.

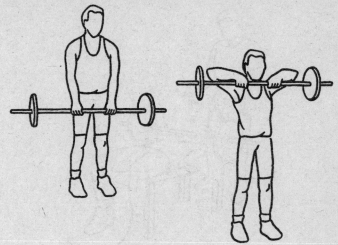

Figure 72. Upright Row

ARM AND CHEST BENCH PRESS

While primarily intended to strengthen the chest and the backs of your arms (triceps), this exercise is also excellent for your wrists.

Lie on your bench, holding a barbell (or dumbbells) with a grip about six inches wider than shoulder-width apart. Keeping the weight to an amount you can control, lower it until it's just about one inch above your midchest. Raise it back in the air, but don't lock your elbows when your arms are extended. Keep your head and hips aligned securely on the bench, and don't arch your back. Do eight to twelve reps, and vary the weight appropriately.

Ankles and Feet

There are two good exercises you can do for this area, which is especially important to focus on if you've had an ankle sprain or two in your past (osteoarthritis is rare in a never-injured ankle).

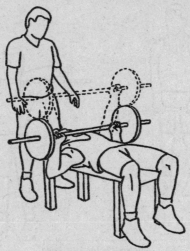

Figure 73. Bench Press

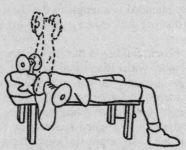

Figure 74. Bench Press

SEATED HEEL RAISE

Sit at the edge of your bench, feet flat on the floor. Hold a barbell or dumbbell on your lower thighs (a few inches up from your knees). Keeping your toes on the ground, lift your heels up as high as they will go, hold them there for five seconds, then gently lower them to the ground. Repeat until you feel your calves and ankles fatigue.

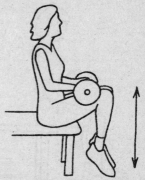

You can make this more difficult by adding more weight, and harder still by putting the full weight on one leg at a time and exercising them separately.

SEATED TOE RAISE

While sitting on the edge of a bench, place one heel on the floor twelve to fifteen inches from the

Figure 75. Seated Heel Raise

bench. Place a five- to ten-pound weight on the top of your shoe, near the toes. You need to hold the weight on your foot with your hand to prevent the weight from slipping off. Keeping your heel on the ground at all times, lift your toes in the air as high as you comfortably can. After eight to twelve repetitions, you may feel fatigue or a slight burning sensation in the front of your shin. This is normal. Switch and do the other foot. If it's more comfortable, place a two- or three-inch lift (a book, a block of wood) under your heel as you perform this exercise.

The above exercises should help you improve the health of certain areas or joints that are particularly problematic. While there are hundreds more we could have added, we believe that providing too many choices can often be counterproductive (particularly if you're just starting to "move" again after a long period of abstinence). Following is a chart to help you plot out your progress on this program and tailor it to meet your needs. Again, make copies and paste to your fridge to mark your progress—and keep you motivated.

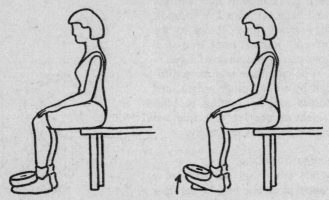

Figure 76. Seated Toe Raise

A Final Thought on Exercise

Exercise can be fun, rewarding, and an excellent outlet for some of the stresses of daily life. So why do so many people who need to exercise avoid it? The problem is often related to lack of motivation or a lack of knowledge of exactly what to do. Some people who want to exercise experience frustration because of the initial effort it takes to get started. They don't think of themselves as ''athletic.'' They often give up before they've given themselves a chance to enjoy the benefits, both physical and psychological. Exercise isn't easy, but we promise you—it gets easier and more enjoyable the longer you keep it up. If you exercise consistently for three months, you'll be hooked. You'll enjoy it. You won't want to quit. And you'll feel far better as a result.

Remember, it's important that you remain active, but don't limit yourself to just one form of exercise. You may need to alter your exercise program midworkout, depending on your symptoms. Pain *is* a good indicator to stop a *particular* movement, but is not an indicator to halt *all* exercise for that day.

STRENGTH TRAINING PROGRESS CHART

	EXERCISES		MON.	TUES.	WED.	THURS.	FRI.	SAT.	SUN.
Exercises for Problem Areas	Knees	Step Up							
		Wall Slide							
		Hamstring Curl							
		Leg Push							
	Hips	Resisted Flexion							
		Resisted Abduction							
		Resisted Adduction							
	Hands and Fingers	Finger Bends							
		Squeeze Ball							
		Finger Extension							
		Agile Finger Stretch							
	Back	"Swimming"							
	Shoulders, Elbows, Wrists	Upright Row							
		Bench Press							
	Ankles and Feet	Seated Heel Raise							
		Seated Toe Raise							

Check the box when you do the exercise.

Imagine, for example, that you are walking on your treadmill and you begin feeling some knee pain. Rather than canceling your workout for the entire day, do an exercise, like stationary biking, that will not hurt the knee. Or move on to working an entirely different body part.

A note about rest. While we are clearly advocates of utilizing the benefits of exercise to combat the negative effects of osteoarthritis, we are also advocates of rest periods between exercise routines. Your success in overcoming osteoarthritis really involves getting to know *your* body and determining a balance between the right amount of exercise and the right amount of rest. Each individual with osteoarthritis is different, and the limitations and abilities he or she experiences vary widely. It's important to remember that the overuse of joints may lead to painful but temporary flare-ups, whereas their underuse may lead to muscle weakness and eventual worsening of your osteoarthritis. It's your personal decision to determine how much exercise—or how little—you should do.

We have given you the basic information you need to create a sensible, individualized program. Once your physical stamina improves, as it will do steadily with this exercise program, and you follow the rest of the arthritis cure, you *will* experience relief, and you will probably be preventing arthritis from striking other areas of your body. So do it for yourself. And don't give up!

6

The Importance of Food and Eating Right

We all know that good nutrition is very important for maintaining a healthy weight and for providing your body with enough energy to get through a busy day. But because of the explosion of interest by both the public and the scientific communities in nutrition and other forms of complementary medicine, we have discovered more about the essential nutritional needs for individuals with injuries and chronic conditions such as osteoarthritis.

To oversimplify for a moment, we now know that there are two interconnected but distinctly different aspects to good nutrition. One has to do with good all-around nutrition—making sure that your diet includes the appropriate amounts of the correct food groups. The other nutritional need is that your diet, in addition to being balanced overall, include foods that contain relatively high levels of the specific nutrients you need to combat your arthritis. Thus, we break this chapter into two sections:

- The first part provides you with a clear understanding of what you need for a healthful overall diet. It demonstrates, by giving you some sample menus and recipes, that sticking to such a diet can be an enjoyable, lifelong experience. You do not need to try to subsist on an extreme diet in order to stay at the right weight and remain energetic and fit. Of course, this book is a total health plan and not an arthritis cookbook. But once you understand your dietary needs, you will have little trouble finding recipes that fulfill them.

• The second part of the chapter summarizes a number of supplementary nutrients you should include in your diet in order to enhance the effects of glucosamine and chondroitin. It also lists the foods that provide those amazing nutrients. (We cover what those substances do, how they work, and how strong the evidence of their effectiveness is in a later chapter.)

A Plan for Successful Eating

The principles of eating correctly are easily understood but hard to live with unless you follow five simple steps:

1. *Plan for your future by creating a nutritional program you can stick to. Don't "diet."* Drastic changes in eating habits just don't "stick." When you lock yourself into an unrealistic, rigid diet, of course you aren't able to adhere to it. In fact, it has been proved beyond a doubt that a conscious restriction of caloric intake is completely ineffective as a long-term weight control method. And yet nearly every one of us sometimes falls prey to the idea that we must "go on a diet" to lose weight. We all know that the weight we lose in this way soon comes back. Yet we still repeat the same mistake. Hope springs eternal—and so, apparently, does diet aid advertising. But the only "diet" that works is a commitment to healthful eating. And that means a commitment to eating healthful foods that you enjoy, and to following a sensible nutritional program that you can live with for the rest of your life. It also means a commitment to eating the right amount—not too much, but also *not too little*. No human being can willingly live on foodstuffs that are boring. And none of us can stick to a diet that leaves us permanently hungry.

The *only* way anyone can stick to a healthful diet is to

make sure it tastes good and satisfies your appetite. The ultimate secret to eating healthfully—and to the food plan we are recommending here—is that *your diet must be tasty and satisfying*. The key is not only to eliminate the "bad" parts of your diet but also to enjoy the new healthful choices you add to replace them.

2. *Set yourself up to succeed.* Make sure your refrigerator, cupboards, pantry shelves, and office contain a variety of tasty, low-fat snacks that are truly satisfying and available when the urge to eat hits. And make sure you don't have any junk food around to tempt you. People who find themselves stressed by life's demands often impulsively reach out for "comfort foods." And it works. There's nothing like a Snickers bar or a doughnut to temporarily lift a miserable mood. Unfortunately, the pleasure lasts only a few moments, but the unneeded weight—and the general lack of wellness that goes with it—seems to last forever.

The problem is that most of us do need the comfort from time to time, and "healthful" snacks don't seem to serve that purpose. So what to do?

The first thing is to be honest with yourself. Don't try to convince yourself that you'll learn to enjoy carrots as much as chocolate. No amount of will power will give you the culinary preferences of a rabbit! Instead, discover a remarkable new world of alternative snacks that don't quite match your current favorites but that are certainly more exciting than carrots. For example, if potato chips, cookies, and ice cream have been your nutritional downfall, replace them with some of the new lines of baked potato chips (which we think taste better than traditional potato chips, and they contain little or no fat); fat-free cookies, brownies, or blondies; or no- or low-fat frozen yogurt. (But remember: Low-fat doesn't mean low-calorie.)

In many cases, initially you will not like the nonfat alternative as much as the "real thing." However, we all know that many of our food and drink preferences are acquired. Few people enjoy beer or coffee the first time they try them. Surprisingly, we can also unacquire tastes. People who used to love fat-laden foods often find that after a few months of not eating any, they dislike foods with high fat contents and genuinely prefer the nonfat foods.

Getting habituated in this way *does* take time, which is probably helpful because, at the same time you are switching to low fat foods, you also want to cut down slightly—*and certainly not increase*—the amount of snacks you consume.

In many ways, you are fortunate if you are making a commitment to healthful eating now because there is such a variety of new nonfat and low-fat foods on the market, with more being added frequently. A word of warning, however: Read the labels carefully.

Nearly all packages for foodstuffs contain a nutritional analysis that includes two key pieces of information: how many grams of fat the food contains, the calories you get from that fat, and the total calories you get from the food. This second piece of information, often ignored, is very important. Let's say that a given food contains 100 calories, and 75 of these are from fat. It may be low in fat, but three-quarters of what you are eating is still fat. It's low compared to 100 percent fat, but it's hardly truly low in fat. This has led to a great deal of confusion, which in turn has led to product labeling laws that give specific definitions to terms such as *low-fat, fat free,* etc. The following table makes clear these definitions.

Fat-Free	Less than ½ gram of fat per serving. (Remember, a package often consists of more than one serving.)
Low-Fat	3 grams of fat or fewer per serving.
Reduced Fat	At least 25 percent less fat than a similar product.
Light or Lite	⅓ less calories or 50 percent less fat.

In regarding the last two categories, always ask yourself, "Reduced from what?" or "Lighter than what?" Labels often say something like, "50 percent less fat than regular doughnuts." Now, regular doughnuts are very high in fat, so high, in fact, that something that has half the fat still has a lot (about 10 grams, down from 20). It's like seeing a Ferrari being sold at half price: $125,000 for a car still isn't cheap!

In addition to reading labels, there are several other tricks to help you eat sensibly during that difficult period when you are retraining your eating habits.

- Pre-prepare sensible portions of snacks so that you aren't tempted to keep eating "because they're there." For example, put single portions of baked potato chips in sandwich bags and then return the sandwich bags to the original bag. When you're ready for your snack, your single portion is already apportioned. But don't be stingy with yourself either. If you make that single portion too small, you'll be tempted to eat more than one bag.

- Prepare the food you plan to cook in advance, when you're not hungry. Have you ever noticed how easy cooking appears when the chef on a TV show whips up a fabulous meal right before your eyes? That's because all the basic food preparation was done in advance. You can do the same; and by doing it when you're not hungry, you will be less likely to snack as you prepare the meal. Once you are hungry, the idea is to prepare the food quickly, get out of the kitchen, and get on with your meal.

3. *Celebrate your eating experience by enhancing your environment.* For instance, rather than eating a frozen microwave dinner right out of the cardboard container, put the fresh food you prepare onto a proper plate and add a variety of vegetables so that your food appeals to your eyes as well as your taste buds. And put on your favorite music while you're at it. The various colors, textures, and smells enhance the dining ambience and go a long way toward enhancing the pleasure and satisfaction of eating. Strangely, if you go to just a little trouble to enjoy the *experience* of eating, you will find yourself less tempted continuously to indulge in the *act* of eating. In other words, you will be inclined to be satisfied with eating less if you enjoy eating more.

On the other hand, if you are dining alone, it is often difficult to motivate yourself to take the trouble to prepare good meals and set the table nicely. But do try. Follow our amended version of the golden rule: "Serve unto yourself what (and how) you would serve unto others."

4. *Eat until you are no longer hungry.* One of the most common poor eating habits that people fall into is to stop eating only when they feel pressure in their stomachs (when they "feel full"), instead of stopping when they feel an end to the "hunger signal" from their brain. Eating until you are no longer "hungry," rather than until you are "full," will put you on the right path to controlling your weight.

5. *Eat slowly.* We know you've heard this advice a hundred times. But it's the best way we know to correctly "hear" your "hunger signal" and therefore stop eating at the right time. Our brains recognize that our stomachs are full rather slowly. If you eat too fast, your brain won't have time to process the information that you've actually had enough to eat. The result: You still feel hungry and therefore continue to eat. If you eat slowly, thereby allowing more time for your brain to receive the "not hungry signal," that feeling of hunger will go away. (We have all heard people complain, "Phew! I ate too much. I feel stuffed." Usually the reason for this is that they ate too quickly.)

Basic Eating Plan

Of course, every one of us is different. We have different tastes, different appetites, different living conditions, and different needs. Obviously, then, each of us needs a different eating plan. In order to provide a plan that everyone can adapt to his or her personal tastes, first we describe the basic food groups that everyone needs, and then we explain how to balance them. This is your basic eating plan.

The purpose of this basic eating plan is to help your arthritis by maximizing the wellness a correct diet generates. While specific foods (which we list later) add nutrients that directly help certain arthritic symptoms, they do you little good if you are not first eating correctly in general.

At the risk of stating the obvious, let us repeat that there are two aspects of eating for good health in general and good joint health in particular: eating a nutritionally balanced menu and maintaining your optimum weight. This latter is especially important for arthritis sufferers because extra weight on already painful joints obviously tends to make them feel worse.

Unfortunately, as we all know, there is no magic diet that causes the pounds to melt off your body, no special combination of foods, no way to juggle proteins, fats, and carbohydrates to ensure weight loss. If there were, everybody would be using it—and losing it. The truth is there is no quick fix. But there *is* an assured slow fix. Simply put, healthful eating leads to heightened energy, which in turn increases your likelihood of sticking to an exercise program—which, in its turn, ultimately helps reduce your osteoarthritic pain. So, briefly, let's review the guidelines for an ideal eating regimen for lifelong good health, as provided by the USDA. It is composed of seven food groupings.

Daily Requirements

1. BREAD, CEREAL, RICE, AND PASTA (6 TO 11 SERVINGS PER DAY) Forming the foundation of a good eating program, these grains are filled with health-enhancing complex carbohydrates, B vitamins, fiber, and other nutrients. A single serving consists of either one slice of bread, 1 ounce of cereal, or ½ cup of cooked rice or pasta.

There are numerous grains to enjoy, including barley, buckwheat, millet, oats, rice, rye, and wheat. Whole grains are more nutritious and have more fiber than processed versions such as white rice or refined flour. So use whole grains whenever possible in your cooking and eating.

2. VEGETABLES (3 TO 5 SERVINGS PER DAY) Low in fat, sodium, and sugar, and with no cholesterol, the vegetable group pro-

vides a variety of vitamins, including A, C, and E, B complex, folic acid, fiber, and various phytochemicals (naturally occurring substances that, while not vitamins or minerals, are necessary for optimal health). For example, the indoles found in broccoli, brussels sprouts, cabbage, and turnips are believed to offer some protection against cancer, as is sulphorophane, a compound also found in these vegetables. Nor should we forget about carotenoids, a group of about six hundred different plant chemicals that help give certain vegetables their color. Known carotenoids, such as alpha- and beta-carotene, B-cryptoxanthin, lutein, capsanthin, and zeaxanthin have been shown to be powerful antioxidants and potential cancer prevention agents. They also are preventive for certain eye diseases, such as macular degeneration (the leading cause of blindness in people over age sixty-five).

A serving of vegetables consists of either 1 cup of raw leafy vegetables, ½ cup of other vegetables (cooked or raw), or ¾ cup of vegetable juice. (Don't include vegetable juice in your diet for more than one serving per day, as it lacks fiber.)

3. FRUIT (2 TO 4 SERVINGS PER DAY)   Like vegetables, fruits are low in fat and sodium, and contain no cholesterol. The fruit group offers vitamin A, B complex, C, fiber, carotenoids, and various phytochemicals, in addition to trace minerals. The elegiac acid in cherries, grapes, and strawberries may "deactivate" certain carcinogens that turn healthy cells cancerous. The glutathione, an antioxidant in avocado, watermelon, and strawberries may help to slow the aging process. And the lycopene in watermelon and tomatoes may help to guard against cancers of the colon, prostate, and bladder.

A single serving of fruit consists of 1 medium fruit, ½ cup fruit cooked or canned in its own juice, or ¾ cup fruit juice. (Only one serving of fruit juice per day should be counted against the total, as it also lacks fiber unless it's the "pulpy" type.)

There are many fruits from which to choose, including apples, apricots, bananas, berries, cantaloupes, cherries, figs, grapefruit, grapes, lemons, limes, mangoes, melons, oranges, papayas, peaches, pears, pineapple, plums, and pomegranates. Learning to pick fruit at its peak is almost an art form. Ask the produce manager at your local market for tips on picking fruit at its peak. Don't give up on a particular fruit unless you've actually tasted it at its best.

4. MEAT, POULTRY, FISH, EGGS, AND DRIED PEAS, BEANS, AND LENTILS (2 TO 3 SERVINGS PER DAY) These "protein" foods provide riboflavin and vitamins B_6 and B_{12}, in addition to other nutrients such as calcium, iron, and niacin, to name a few, and, of course, protein. When eating red meat, look for lean cuts and cut away any visible fat. If you eat poultry, remember that white meat gets only 15 percent of its calories from fat, whereas darker meat gets more than 30 percent.

Many varieties of fish, such as brook trout, cod, flounder, haddock, halibut, red snapper, sea bass, tuna (packed in water), and yellow perch, tend to be lower in fat. Norway sardines, salmon, shellfish, Atlantic mackerel, pink salmon, and sablefish contain more fat, but much of the fat they do contain consists of the "good" omega-3 fatty acids, which can help to reduce the risk of coronary heart disease, and the inflammation in rheumatoid arthritis.

Peas, beans, and lentils, collectively called legumes, are an overlooked and very health-enhancing source of protein. They have no cholesterol and are low in fat, sugar, and sodium. They contain vitamins B_1 and B_6, calcium, fiber, complex carbohydrates, phytochemicals, and other nutrients.

A single serving consists of 2–3 ounces of cooked, lean meat, poultry, or fish, or ½ cup cooked dried beans. (Note: 1 egg counts as 1 ounce of lean meat).

5. MILK, YOGURT, AND CHEESES (2 TO 3 SERVINGS PER DAY) These foods offer protein, calcium, vitamin D, and other nutrients necessary for strong bones and connective tissues. Choose the low-fat or nonfat varieties whenever possible. (After a reasonable habituation period, 1 percent and then nonfat milk tastes every bit as good as 2 percent milk.)

A single serving consists of either 1 cup milk, 1½ ounces

of natural cheese, 2 ounces of processed cheese, or 1 (6 ounces) cup of yogurt.

6. SWEETS AND ALCOHOLIC BEVERAGES   You obviously cannot do without any sweets altogether (at least, very, very few of us are able to). And many people are unwilling to cut out alcohol entirely. The rule on both these foodstuffs is to keep them to a minimum. To the extent that you do consume them, cut down on your intake of grain servings to compensate. But whenever you can, substitute whole grains for "liquid" ones.

7. FATS AND OILS   These foods offer little nutritional value and are high in calories. Remember to use olive oil as your main cooking fat. As a substitute, consider using juices instead of butter or oils when sautéing vegetables. Doing this provides a delicious way of enhancing a food's flavor, while reducing the addition of unnecessary fat. If you have an inflammatory joint problem, there is a place for supplementing your diet with certain anti-inflammatory oils, such as GLA and EPA. Fortunately, these supplements will not contribute to a significant number of excess calories.

Putting It All Together

To summarize, a simple yet powerfully effective diet is based on these commonsense recommendations:

- 6–11 grain servings per day
- 3–5 vegetable servings per day
- 2–4 fruit servings per day
- 2–3 "protein" servings per day
- 2–3 dairy servings per day
- As little sugar as you can manage
- As little fat as you can manage

In regards to these last two points, remember that all protein-rich and most other foods—except nearly all fruits and vegetables—contain at least some fat, so there is generally no danger that you'll get too little of it. Similarly, so many foods contain sugar that if you never ate sweets at all, you would still be getting more than you need.

The number of servings you need depends on how large and how active you are. While there is no absolute rule here, because every one of us is different, there are some guidelines:

Food Group	Servings per Day	Sedentary Women and Some Older Men	Active Women and Many Sedentary Men	Active Men and Some Very Active Women
Grain	6–11	6	9	11
Vegetable	3–5	3	4	5
Fruit	2–4	2	3	4
Protein	2–3	2	2	3
Dairy	2–3	2–3	2–3	2–3

A Sample Menu

Before we move on, it's time to prove to you that there is absolutely no need to commit yourself to a bland or boring diet. ''Good for you'' food can be downright exciting.

To give you an idea of just how good it can be, just consider the following day's menu, the sort of day you would plan if you had special guests staying for breakfast, lunch, and dinner! Yes, it's completely in line with our nutritional guidelines, and all you need to do to accommodate your particular needs (based on the degree of activity in your daily life) is to adjust the size of the portions. Sure, this menu is a bit labor intensive to prepare, but we want to show you first how *delicious* truly healthy food can taste. Later, we show you that it can be easy, too.

· A GOURMET BREAKFAST ·

Almost Danish

A real Danish provides little nutrition but lots of fat, sugar, and calories. This Danish is just the opposite, and it tastes excellent.

3 plain bagels, split in half
1 cup part-skim ricotta cheese
3 teaspoons honey
¾ teaspoon cinnamon

Toast bagels very lightly. Mix together ricotta cheese, honey, and cinnamon. Spread equal amounts on all the bagel halves. Broil cheese-covered bagels for 1 to 2 minutes, or until cheese mixture melts. Makes 6 servings.

1 pint of fresh strawberries, rinsed well. Remove tops and serve. Makes 6 servings.

The best coffee money can buy (stick to one cup with sugar substitute and nonfat milk, if we can't persuade you to be a real coffee connoisseur and take it black!).

· AN ELEGANT LUNCH ·

ONION-LEMON FISH

This is a palate-pleasing way to prepare just about any kind of fish. Make sure you select a white fish such as rock cod, sea bass, or snapper and that the pieces are well formed and uniform in size and color.

>   2 medium-sweet Spanish onions (8–10 oz. each)
>   1 large lemon, thinly sliced, seeds removed
>   2 cups water
>   ½ cup white wine
>   1 bay leaf
>   ¼ teaspoon whole peppercorns
>   ¼ teaspoon salt
>   1½ pounds fish fillets
>   ⅓ cup plain nonfat yogurt
>   1 teaspoon chopped fresh dill weed

Slice onions into ¼" slices. Arrange onion and lemon slices in a large nonstick skillet. Add water, wine, bay leaf, peppercorns, and salt. Bring to a boil. Cover and simmer for 10 minutes. Remove an onion and a lemon slice for each piece of fish and set aside.

Place fish fillets on top of the remaining onion and lemon slices in the skillet. They should be about a third to half covered in the poaching liquid. If necessary, add a touch more wine. Top each fillet with the reserved slice of onion and lemon. Cover skillet and simmer fish for 5 to 8 minutes or until it flakes with a fork. Do not overcook. Remove skillet from heat.

Prepare the accompanying sauce by combining the yogurt

and dill with 1 tablespoon of the poaching liquid. Season to taste with salt and pepper. Remove fish from liquid to a plate and garnish with the onions and lemons from the skillet, as well as fresh dill weed. Serve with yogurt sauce. Makes 6 servings.

Brown Rice Parmigiana

A great accompaniment to fish, poultry, or meat. Don't overdo it on the Parmesan cheese, though, since it's high in both sodium and fat. In any case, too much of it detracts from the delicate flavor of the fish.

3 shallots, finely chopped
¾ cup zucchini, diced
1 small garlic clove, minced
¾ cup chopped onions
3 cups chicken broth
1½ cups uncooked brown rice
2 tablespoons (flat, not heaping) grated Parmesan cheese

In a nonstick frying pan, sauté shallots, zucchini, garlic, and onions in a few tablespoons of chicken broth. Add rice and continue to sauté until rice begins to crackle. Bring remaining chicken broth to a boil in a separate pot and add to rice/vegetable mixture in frying pan. Reduce heat to simmer, cover, and cook for 45 minutes or until all the liquid has been absorbed. Toss with Parmesan cheese and serve. Makes 6 servings.

ASPARAGUS BELGIQUE

This dish does double duty—either as a side dish or as a salad.

36 spears of asparagus, cooked and chilled
½ teaspoon powdered mustard
½ teaspoon grated lemon peel
3 tablespoons rice vinegar
2 tablespoons lemon juice
1 teaspoon olive oil
1 tablespoon water
dash salt
dash pepper
2 tablespoons pimiento, chopped

Place asparagus in a shallow dish. Combine all other ingredients except the pimiento in a blender and blend well. Pour mixture over asparagus. Top with pimiento. Cover and refrigerate for 1 to 2 hours. Makes 4–6 servings.

STRAWBERRIES ROMANOFF

As if Onion-Lemon Fish with Brown Rice Parmigiana and Asparagus Belgique weren't enough elegance for one luncheon . . .

4 tablespoons dry white wine
3 tablespoons frozen orange juice concentrate, thawed
3 cups sliced strawberries, stems removed
¾ cup low-fat frozen dairy whipped topping, thawed

In a medium bowl, combine wine and orange juice. Add strawberries and toss well to coat. Cover with plastic wrap and refrigerate for 1 to 2 hours.

When ready to serve, divide strawberry mixture evenly into 6 dessert dishes. Top each portion with 2 tablespoons whipped topping. Makes 6 delectable servings.

CRACKED WHEAT BREAD

This is a dense, heavy bread worthy of being called "the staff of life." It's particularly good with a hearty soup, like minestrone, but we like it with just about anything. (It's fun baking bread. But obviously you don't have to make your own if you don't want to. You can buy an excellent version of this at many stores. Just make sure that the bread you purchase is whole grain and contains little fat.)

> 2 cakes compressed yeast
> ¾ cup lukewarm water
> 2 tablespoons olive oil
> 2 tablespoons honey
> 3 cups cooked cracked wheat
> 1 teaspoon salt
> 6 cups whole wheat flour

Dissolve yeast in warm water and set aside for 10 minutes. Grease a large bowl with 1 tablespoon of the olive oil so that it's ready to receive the dough, and dust a kneading board with flour. Put the yeasty water, the rest of the oil, honey, cracked wheat, and salt into a mixing bowl. Gradually add the whole wheat flour, 1 cup at a time, mixing until smooth.

Turn out onto the floured board and knead for about 5 minutes. Place in the oiled bowl, turning so that the top of the dough gets lightly covered, and allow to rise until approximately double in size.

Punch down, form into two loaves, and put into greased bread pans (use a very quick spray of Pam, or a similar product, or just a touch of olive oil). Allow to rise again until doubled. Bake at 400° for about 1 hour. Makes 2 loaves, each containing about 8 slices approximately 1" thick.

Eat one slice as soon as the bread has cooled. This is the baker's rightful reward and therefore contains absolutely no calories . . . however, a second slice contains *double* the calories, so beware!

· AN AFTERNOON GOURMET SNACK ·

For a terrific snack. . . .

MINESTRONE SOUP

This is a great recipe, just like Mom used to make. If you have any vegetables in the house that aren't listed in this recipe, feel free to throw them in. (Mom always did!)

Of course, you don't want to make this soup every day. Make a big batch every few weeks and freeze it in individual containers, then thaw as required. People often don't think of soup as a snack, but it's ideal: easy to make without being high in calories, and you can make it into quite an elegant presentation.

>   *1 cup dried beans*
>   *3 cups water*
>   *6 bouillon cubes*
>   *1 cup broccoli or cauliflower florets*
>   *1 cup onions, chopped*
>   *1 cup shredded spinach or cabbage*
>   *1 cup carrots, finely diced*
>   *1 cup fresh green beans*
>   *1 cup celery, chopped*
>   *1 tablespoon minced garlic*
>   *½ cup finely chopped parsley*
>   *1 medium zucchini, diced*
>   *¼ teaspoon dried rosemary*
>   *2 tablespoons fresh basil (or 1 tablespoon dried)*

1/4 teaspoon pepper
2 cups tomato juice
1 cup whole-wheat macaroni, uncooked

Soak beans overnight in water. Drain and place in a pot with 3 cups of fresh water, plus bouillon cubes. Cover and simmer for 1 hour. Drain, reserving cooking water. In a blender, blend half the beans with 2 cups of the cooking water. Set aside with the remaining beans and the remaining cooking water.

In another pot, use the remaining cooking water to water-sauté the vegetables and spices until tender. Add tomato juice, blended beans, and reserved whole beans. Bring to a boil. Lower heat and simmer for 1 hour. Add macaroni and simmer for an additional 15 minutes, or until macaroni is tender. Makes 12 one-cup servings.

Serve soup with 1 slice of Cracked Wheat Bread (see page 160). There, who said a snack can't be an occasion?

· A FINE DINNER ·

While you really do want to keep it light, if lunch was elegant, then surely dinner must be sumptuous. The answer, of course, is chicken. As Coq au Vin, Thai Tipsy Chicken, or Poulet Rôti, the good ol' hen can take on any number of haute cuisine mantles. This evening, you will make one of the best: Crispy Crunchy Chicken.

CRISPY CRUNCHY CHICKEN

This is a delightful, slimmed down advance over anything the Colonel ever conceived. And it's easy to cook (which is just as well, since you've been cooking all day).

    2 cups wheat germ
    2 teaspoons dried tarragon leaves, finely crushed
    2 teaspoons grated lemon peel
    ½ cup skim milk
    2 three-pound chickens, cut up and skinned

Combine wheat germ, tarragon, and lemon peel in a shallow container. Stir well to blend. Pour milk into another shallow container and dip chicken pieces first into milk, then into wheat germ mixture, coating evenly. Place chicken pieces on a foil-lined pan. Bake at 375° for 45 to 50 minutes. Makes 8 servings. (Leftovers are delicious for lunch tomorrow.)

PILAF OF WILD RICE AND MUSHROOMS

Wild rice (which isn't really a rice at all—it's a great-tasting grass) makes a luxurious side dish, and it goes very well with the crunch of your chicken.

    3 quarts water
    1½ cups wild rice
    1½ cups fresh mushrooms, sliced
    ½ cup dry white wine
    1½ cups chicken or beef broth
    4 tablespoons finely minced carrot
    ½ teaspoon dried thyme
    5 tablespoons finely minced onion
    4 tablespoons finely minced celery
    ½ teaspoon ground pepper
    2 bay leaves

Preheat oven to 350°. Bring water to a boil and add rice. Boil uncovered for 5 minutes. Drain rice.

In a medium skillet, sauté the vegetables and spices in the white wine and broth until tender. Add the rice and cook over high heat for 1 minute.

Put mixture into a casserole dish and bake at 350° for 35

minutes or until rice is tender. Check periodically while baking to see if mixture has gone dry. If so, add a few drops of broth. Remove bay leaves before serving. Makes 4 servings.

STEAMED VEGETABLES WITH WHITE WINE SAUCE

You want vegetables and you don't want them to be boring. But who needs fatty cream sauces? This white wine sauce is a perfect addition to any fish, chicken, or vegetable dish. We've chosen broccoli, but you can use this sauce with most any vegetable you prefer. It will add the finishing gourmet touch to this evening's entrée.

1½ cups nonfat milk
1½ tablespoons cornstarch
2 shallots, minced
2 tablespoons dry white wine
6 cups broccoli florets, steamed

Mix 3 tablespoons of the milk with the cornstarch and set aside. Bring the remaining milk to a boil in a small saucepan. When it starts to foam, reduce the heat to a simmer. Gradually add a little of the hot milk to the cornstarch paste, thinning it more and more until it mixes easily with the milk without lumps. Return milk/cornstarch mixture to the saucepan, add shallots and white wine, and cook over medium heat until thickened, stirring constantly. Pour over precooked broccoli and serve. Makes 6 servings.

BANANAS FLAMBÉ

A low-fat version of the high-class favorite.

3 large bananas, split lengthwise
¾ cup apple juice

Generous dash of cinnamon
¾ teaspoon vanilla extract
½ teaspoon grated lemon rind
½ teaspoon ground ginger
3 tablespoons brandy
6 scoops frozen vanilla yogurt, or substitute your favorite flavor

Place banana halves in a nonstick frying pan. Add apple juice, cinnamon, vanilla, lemon rind, and ginger and cook over low heat for 3 to 5 minutes, continually basting bananas with the juice. Heat the brandy in a small pot, then pour over the bananas. Ignite the brandy and carefully shake the pan until the flames die out. Serve immediately, one half banana topped with one scoop of frozen yogurt per person. Makes 6 servings.

We're sure you will agree that this has been a gourmet day. But it also has been one with a carefully balanced diet. Here is the nutritional summary of what you have eaten.

Nutritional Information

Food Group	Servings per Day	Breakfast	Lunch	Snack	Dinner	Total
Grain	6–11	x	xx	x	xx	6
Vegetable	3–5		x	x	x	3
Fruit	2–4	x	x		x	3
Protein	2–3		x	x	x	3
Dairy	2–3	x	x		x	3

See, it's easy! You can eat wonderful and elegant food all day long and still stay solidly within your diet. By eating healthfully, you don't have to compromise on quality or feel deprived.

Of course, unless you are a truly dedicated cook, you won't

go to this much trouble every day. Fortunately, cooking doesn't have to be particularly time-consuming, and healthful cooking takes no longer than any other kind. So allow us to give you two examples of fast, delicious, healthful, full-day menus. As you read them, you'll see at once that they are in no way difficult to make or spartan in content. On the contrary, they're easy and delicious. And when you read their nutritional content, you'll see that they are also properly nutritionally balanced.

The first menu is an example for a typical day, not overly elegant, not overly rushed. The second is one where you're rushed off your feet. That happens to all of us, but it doesn't mean we cannot eat a healthful and tasty diet.

Sample Menu for a Typical Day's Healthful Eating

Okay, let's start with a "standard" day. Remember to make the appropriate portion modifications based on how active a lifestyle you lead.

· BREAKFAST ·

FRUITY MILKSHAKE

A fast but nutritious way to start the day.

    1 cup nonfat milk
    4 tablespoons plain nonfat yogurt
    ½ teaspoon vanilla extract
    1 ripe banana, papaya, or mango, or 1 whole peach (pitted)
    1 teaspoon cinnamon
    ¼ teaspoon nutmeg

Place all ingredients into a blender and blend until smooth. Makes 1 to 2 servings.

BLUEBERRY BRAN MUFFIN

We often buy low-fat muffins at our local gourmet store. They are excellent, and they are "fat-free," which means that they contain less than half a gram of fat each. However, if you have time, you can easily bake these at home. They keep for several days when refrigerated in a baggie and much longer when frozen. (Each muffin counts as 2 grain servings.)

1 cup stone-ground whole-wheat flour
1 cup undiluted defrosted apple juice concentrate
1 teaspoon baking soda
1¾ cups unprocessed bran
¾ cup nonfat milk
½ teaspoon cinnamon
1 cup fresh or frozen (unsweetened) blueberries
½ teaspoon ground cloves
½ teaspoon ground nutmeg
1 egg white
½ teaspoon vanilla extract

Preheat oven to 350°. Mix together all ingredients, making sure to stir until the batter is smooth. Pour into a greased muffin tin and bake for 20 minutes, until a toothpick inserted in a muffin's center comes out clean. Makes 1 dozen small muffins.

Coffee or tea (with skim milk and sweetener, if desired).

· LUNCH ·

CHICKEN SALAD RIVIERA

The combination of chicken, curry, raisins, and almonds makes this salad both exotic and delicious—yet light enough so that it won't slow you down. And it takes only a few minutes to prepare.

> 1 20-ounce can of pineapple chunks (packed in their own juice)
> ¼ cup raisins
> ¼ cup slivered almonds
> 12 ounces cooked breast of chicken, cut into 1-inch chunks
> 3 tablespoons sliced green onion
> ¼ cup cooked green peas
> ¼ cup sliced celery
> Curry Dressing (see below)
> Salad greens, to garnish

Drain pineapple of its juice. Then combine all ingredients in a large bowl. Toss with Curry Dressing and serve on salad plates lined with crisp greens. Makes 4 servings.

CURRY DRESSING

You can make a lot extra if you like. It will keep for a couple of weeks in the refrigerator, and it's delicious over fruit, as a dip, or as dressing on green salads.

> 1 cup plain nonfat yogurt
> 2 tablespoons honey

2 teaspoons fresh lime juice
1 teaspoon curry powder
Dash of salt

Combine all ingredients. Blend well. Makes 4 servings, ¼ cup each.

Add 2 slices of cracked wheat bread (page 160) and diet soda or mineral water and the meal is complete.

· MIDAFTERNOON SNACK ·

SPICED POPCORN

We recommend a midafternoon snack. It keeps you from getting so hungry that you overeat at night. Popcorn is one of the world's most nutritious snacks and, when properly prepared, it's also one of the lowest in fat.

¼ teaspoon salt
2 tablespoons tomato paste
½ teaspoon chili powder
2 tablespoons water
½ teaspoon olive oil
½ teaspoon garlic powder
8 cups air-popped popcorn

Preheat oven to 250°. Combine all ingredients except for the popcorn, in a small glass container (such as a custard cup) and microwave for 30 seconds, or until mixture bubbles. Pour over popcorn and toss to coat thoroughly. Spread coated popcorn on a jelly roll pan and bake until dry, about 2 or 3 minutes. Makes 4 servings.

You can add raw vegetables and an apple to your snack

to make it into a truly satisfying near-meal or you can have a cup of nonfat milk or a single serving of nonfat yogurt.

· DINNER ·

YEMENITE DELIGHT

You can make this dish with any white meat, including chicken, veal, pork loin, ostrich (which is very low in fat but not in price), turkey breast, etc. With the exotic aromas of this dish, you'll feel as if you've been transported to a sultan's palace!

1 teaspoon olive oil
4 pieces of white meat about 3 ounces each (all fat cut
    off, and skin removed)
1 onion, chopped
3 carrots, peeled and sliced diagonally
½ teaspoon cinnamon
¼ teaspoon salt
¼ teaspoon paprika
¼ teaspoon ground ginger
1 teaspoon curry powder
Pinch of cardamom
1½ cups chicken broth
¾ cup bulgur wheat or rice, uncooked
1 green pepper, sliced in ¼-inch strips

Heat oil in a large, heavy skillet. Add meat and brown lightly on both sides. Remove meat from skillet.

Add onion, carrots, and spices to skillet and sauté until onions are golden brown. If there is not enough liquid, add a little chicken broth. Stir in remaining chicken broth and bulgur or rice. Place the pieces of meat on top of the bulgur or rice and place the green pepper strips over the meat. Cover and simmer for about 30 minutes, or until the meat is tender and the bulgur or rice has absorbed all of the broth. Makes 4 servings.

Nutritional Information

Food Group	Servings per Day	Breakfast	Lunch	Snack	Dinner	Total
Grain	6–11	xx	xx		xx	6
Vegetable	3–5		xx	x	xx	5
Fruit	2–4	x	xx	x		4
Protein	2–3	x	x		x	3
Dairy	2–3	x		x		2

As you can see, this day's tasty menu is well balanced. This is an example of the quantity and number of servings per day that are reasonable for someone trying to reach their ideal weight. Of course exercise is a big component in achieving that goal.

When You're Rushed off Your Feet

This is one of those days where you barely have time to think, let alone cook meals. You'll be eating on the run. Even so, there's no need to eat two candy bars for lunch. Here's an example of a healthful alternative. (Again, remember to make the necessary adjustments to take your lifestyle and needs into account.)

• BREAKFAST •

• 1 cup cereal with nonfat milk (choose a nonfat, high-fiber cereal, such as raisin bran)

- 1 bagel with jam, honey, or nonfat cream cheese (no butter)
- 1 eight-oz. glass of orange juice
- Nutritional protein bar or drink
- Coffee or tea, with skim milk and sweetener, if desired (optional).

· LUNCH ·

OPEN-FACE VEGGIE DELIGHT

2–4 teaspoons Dijon mustard
Whole-grain English muffin, split and toasted
½ cup broccoli florets
¼ cup chopped red, green, and/or yellow bell pepper
¼ cup shredded carrots
½ cup grated low-fat Monterey Jack cheese

Preheat your oven's broiler. Spread mustard on split sides of each muffin. Arrange veggies on top, then sprinkle on the cheese. Place in broiler, about four inches from heat for two to three minutes or until cheese melts.

Fresh salad (the darker shade of green the lettuce, the better) with a very low-fat or nonfat dressing, or a squeeze of lemon juice from a freshly cut wedge.

1 glass nonfat milk.

· SNACK ·

JUICE POPS

These frozen fruit bars are just the thing during the dog days of summer! Premake for a refreshing vitamin C–filled snack in a second.

  1¼ cup pineapple juice or orange juice
  ¼ cup undiluted orange juice concentrate, defrosted
  ½ cup crushed pineapple or 1 ripe banana or 4 large
      strawberries, sliced
  ¼ cup plain nonfat yogurt

Combine all ingredients in a blender and blend until smooth. Fill pop molds or ice cube trays with the mixture and freeze until firm. Makes 8 pops.

You can stretch your snack by adding two or three crackers or a slice of low-fat whole-grain bread.

· DINNER ·

SALMON CROQUETTES

Delicious and so easy! These croquettes take only 20 minutes, and most of that is cooking time, when you can be setting the table or whatever else needs doing. However, this recipe tastes as if you really slaved! (Croquettes can be made in advance and frozen.)

Nonstick cooking spray
1 sixteen-oz. can water-packed salmon, drained
½ cup dry plain bread crumbs
½ cup chopped celery
½ cup chopped onion
¼ cup liquid egg substitute or 1 egg white
2 tablespoons chopped parsley
2 teaspoons lemon juice
¼ teaspoon celery seed
¼ teaspoon white pepper
¼ teaspoon garlic powder

Preheat your oven to 375°. Spray a cookie sheet with nonstick vegetable cooking spray. Combine all the ingredients in a medium-size bowl. Mix well. Shape salmon mixture into 6 patties. Arrange on a large cookie sheet.

Bake at 375° for 10 minutes. Turn over and bake 5 more minutes until warmed through and crisp. Makes 6 servings. Serve with a slice of Cracked Wheat Bread (page 160).

Nutritional Information

Food Group	Servings per Day	Breakfast	Lunch	Snack	Dinner	Total
Grain	6–11	xx	xx	x	x	6
Vegetable	3–5		xxx			3
Fruit	2–4	x		x		2
Protein	2–3	x			x	2
Dairy	2–3	x	x			2

We figure you've spent a total of half an hour cooking all day long. Add another twenty mintues serving and cleaning up. We think it's worth that much time to make sure you're eating properly. And, as you see, this is again at the lower end of the recommended daily consumption level. Yet there's plenty to eat. If you're of average size and do an ordinary amount of activities, you won't feel hungry and deprived.

Obviously, all three menus assume that you cook at home. But of course you may be working or otherwise out of the house. Or you may just be eating out for fun. Or maybe you just hate to cook. In those circumstances, there are temptations to eat inappropriately. We never said that eating correctly doesn't require some will power! But if you want to, you certainly can stick to a sensible diet away from home. Even fast-food places almost always serve *some* low-fat meals. And certainly most good restaurants do. Just look the waiter in the eye and *demand* that your food be grilled without oil. And send it back if he "forgets"!

You should be aware that most of the larger chains are willing to provide you with the dietary analysis of the food they serve. All you have to do is ask. Or you can visit Brenda Adderly's Web site at www.BrendaAdderly.com to obtain that information, as well as additional tasty recipes.

Nutrients Helpful to Maximizing the Arthritis Cure— and How to Get Them

Now we'd like to move forward to discuss the specific nutrients you should be trying to obtain from your diet. In chapter 7 we'll tell you how to further maximize the arthritis cure by adding other supplementary nutrients to glucosamine and chondroitin, which you should be taking daily. You can, of course, add these nutrients by taking multivitamins and multimineral supplements in pill form. We give a clear prescription for you to do this in that chapter. Though the supplements are important, you still need to make sure that most of your nutrients are obtained by eating food. Food provides nutrients not found in supplements, including certain plant chemicals, fibers, and perhaps dozens of important substances we have yet to discover.

The following describes the best way to obtain a wide variety of nutrients through food sources. To start, we'll provide a list of nutrients known to complement the beneficial effect of glucosamine and chondroitin in order to maximize the arthritis cure. They fall into four categories:

- Minerals your body needs for its enzymes to function optimally and thus maximize the impact of chondroitin and glucosamine
- Antioxidants with which to neutralize the ''scavenger'' radicals that speed the degeneration of cartilage
- Bioflavonoids, which enhance the ability of collagen to build and maintain strong cartilage and also have antioxidant properties
- Vitamin D, which seems to slow the progression of osteoarthritis

We consider these one at a time and provide you with a listing of the foodstuffs that contain them. You will see that those foods can easily be incorporated into your daily diet.

Minerals

There are five main trace minerals that are known to be important adjuncts to the arthritis cure, two additional trace minerals that may also be helpful, and two other minerals you need in larger quantities. You should ingest all of them—and the foods that are especially rich in these minerals—daily.

If you look carefully at the list, the only foods you need regularly are ones that fit neatly into almost any balanced menu:

- Green vegetables, especially broccoli
- Some legumes
- Milk
- Potatoes
- Whole grains
- Dried fruit (prunes, raisins, and dates)

Antioxidants

The basic antioxidants your body needs are easy to remember: vitamins A, C, and E and the mineral selenium. As a mne-

Nutrients Helpful to Maximizing
the Arthritis Cure

		FOODS
Minerals	Boron	Grapes
		Plums
		Dried fruit
		Leafy vegetables
		Nuts
		Grains
	Chromium	Broccoli
		Mushrooms
		Wheat germ
		Beef
		Chicken
		Seafood
		Dairy products
		Potatoes w/ skin
		Fresh fruit
	Manganese	Whole grains
		Peas
		Spinach
		Nuts and peanuts
		Avocados
		Blackberries
		Pineapple
		Egg yolks
		Dried beans
	Selenium	Broccoli
		Cabbage
		Celery
		Cucumbers
		Garlic
		Mushrooms
		Onions

Nutrients Helpful to Maximizing the Arthritis Cure (continued)

Minerals	Selenium (cont'd)	Chicken
		Whole grain
		Bran
		Egg yolk
		Seafood
		Milk
	Zinc	Grains
		Nuts
		Seeds
		Red meat
		Potatoes
		Oysters
		Seafood
		Poultry
		Milk
		Soybeans
		Eggs
		Mushrooms
	Copper	Legumes
		Potatoes
		Oysters/shellfish
		Soybeans
		Nuts
		Salmon
		Barley
		Mushrooms
		Oatmeal
	Silicon	Potatoes
		Cereal
		Apples
		Brown rice
		Seafood
		Soybeans

Nutrients Helpful to Maximizing the Arthritis Cure (*continued*)

Minerals	Silicon (cont'd)	Beets
		Green, leafy veggies
Minerals	Calcium	Milk and other dairy
		Whole grains
		Shrimp
		Salmon
		Green leafy vegetables
		Brazil nuts
		Almonds
		Broccoli
		Tofu
		Oysters
		Cabbage
		Asparagus
		Sesame seeds
		Carob
	Magnesium	Green vegetables
		Soybeans
		Halibut
		Shrimp
		Swordfish
		Cod
		Fruit juice
		Nuts
		Milk
		Peaches
		Apricots
Anti-oxidants	Vitamin A (and its precursor Beta-Carotene)	Milk
		Cheese
		Eggs
		Liver
		Turkey
		Carrots

Nutrients Helpful to Maximizing
the Arthritis Cure (*continued*)

Anti-oxidants	Vitamin A (and its precursor Beta-Carotene) (cont.)	Sweet potatoes
		Broccoli
		Spinach
		Tomatoes
		Watermelon
		Cantaloupe
		Apricots
		Papaya
		Pumpkin
	Vitamin C	Oranges
		Grapefruit
		Cantaloupe
		Strawberries
		Parsley
		Spinach
		Bananas
		Tomatoes
		Cabbage
		Broccoli
		Red pepper
		Papaya
		Kiwi
	Vitamin E	Asparagus
		Avocado
		Broccoli
		Peanut Butter
		Sunflower Seeds
		Whole Grain Bread

monic, we call them the four ACES. These essentials are widely available in foodstuffs.

- *Vitamin A* is found in milk, liver, and turkey. There's also the "plant form" of vitamin A, the carotenoids (the phyto-chemicals we mentioned earlier). They are found in apricots, carrots, cantaloupe, papayas, peaches, pumpkin, and all yellow-orange fruits and vegetables, as well as in dark green leafy vegetables such as broccoli, spinach, and parsley. A few of the six hundred major carotenoids, alpha- and beta-carotenes and beta-cryptoxanthin, can actually be converted into vitamin A in the body. In addition to augmenting the maximizing effects of the arthritis cure, vitamin A encourages fertility, promotes the secretion of "digestive juices," and helps to keep the linings of the colon, esophagus, gall-bladder, kidneys, intestine, stomach, rectum, and urinary tract intact.
- *Vitamin C* is found in a variety of foods, including oranges, parsley, grapefruit, cantaloupe, bananas, tomatoes, cabbage, broccoli, red peppers, papaya, and kiwi. In addition to aiding the arthritis cure, this vitamin is necessary for a strong immune system, iron absorption, regulation of cholesterol levels, healthy capillaries, and production of cartilage components, proteoglycans, and collagen.
- *Vitamin E* is found in asparagus, avocados, broccoli, peanut butter, almonds, hazelnuts, sunflower seeds, wheat germ, dried prunes, vegetable oils, and whole-grain breads and cereals. In addition to guarding against free-radical damage, vitamin E helps keep the immune system strong and may be an important aid in fighting cancer. Scientists who conducted early research on vitamin E noted that its absence from food made laboratory rats sterile. In recognition of this fact, they named it tocopherol, which means "to bring forth children." However, just plain old vitamin E may not do the trick; there is some evidence to suggest that the best vitamin E supplements may have a combination of two or more forms of the vitamin, at least alpha- and gamma-tocopherol. These occur

naturally in the foods noted, but if you buy vitamin E in a jar, make sure you are getting the combination.
- *Selenium* is found in whole grains, wheat germ, nuts, poultry, fish, and meat, and in lesser amounts in fruits and vegetables such as cabbage, broccoli, celery, cucumbers, garlic, and mushrooms. The amount of selenium in fruits and vegetables varies considerably, depending on how much was in the soil in which the foods were grown.

Bioflavonoids

These are special nutrients that are important for overall health and for helping to enhance the effects of the arthritis cure. Flavonoids are found in green vegetables and are concentrated in the skins of fruits. They are also in tea, coffee, and wine.

Vitamin D

There are two forms of vitamin D, one which is found in some of the foods we eat, and the other manufactured by our bodies when exposed to sunlight. Vitamin D is fat-soluble, and can thus build up inside the body. As a result, it can be highly toxic when taken in large doses for an extended period of time. Vitamin D is important in that it helps in the development of strong bones. The most common source of vitamin D is fortified milk. Other sources include herring, sardines, salmon, and cod liver oil.

(We explain more fully how they work in Chapter 7.)

In Summary

There you have it. We hope you agree that it is truly not very hard to adhere to an eating pattern that maintains a balance of nutritional ingredients and adds those special foods that are particularly valuable to people with osteoarthritis. One thing we can promise you: If you do follow this fairly simple program and stick to it, your osteoarthritis will be improved, your general health will be enhanced, and you will live a much fuller and happier life.

7

The Maximizing Supplement Plan—and New Developments That May Enhance the Effectiveness of Glucosamine and Chondroitin

A lot has happened since we first wrote *The Arthritis Cure*. Laboratories worldwide have reported on exciting new studies that support the early promise of glucosamine and chondroitin sulfates (see Appendix A for the latest findings) and other nutritional substances and minerals have shown that they may add to the impact of glucosamine and chondroitin to achieve an even quicker and more complete treatment. The purpose of this chapter is to provide you with the latest information on additional supplements that can maximize the efficacy of glucosamine and chondroitin—and thus maximize healing.

We'll also provide a simple program which, followed regularly, can lead to faster, stronger healing at any stage of the cure.

The Importance of Supplements in Addition to a Healthful Diet

One of the most significant new developments in the treatment of osteoarthritis is the use of minerals and trace minerals, which the body requires for normal functioning. A large percentage of the population is deficient in at least one, and often several, of these minerals. Trace minerals are needed in very small amounts, in *thousandths or millionths* of a gram (a gram being about one twenty-eighth of an ounce) and are required components of most enzymes. Enzymes, in turn, are required for almost all chemical reactions in the body, including those involved with cartilage repair.

Minerals are available in food (mainly fruits and vegetables) or supplement form. We recommended in Chapter 6 that you eat a wide variety of foods, especially fruits and vegetables, in order to ensure that you get enough vitamins, minerals, and phytochemicals to stay healthy. Eating healthfully is required to ensure that your body has all of the necessary ingredients to create a healing environment. But sometimes good nutrition is not enough, and it's a shame to hinder your own natural repair system by simply being deficient in one or two nutrients, especially if those nutrients are easy to obtain.

The National Research Council established the RDAs (recommended daily allowances) needed of each nutrient. They maintain that the RDAs can be obtained by eating a well-balanced diet, without the use of supplements. There's a big difference, however, between getting your RDAs, and *getting enough of these nutrients to treat or prevent osteoarthritis*. That's why we believe that, for arthritis sufferers, there are some limitations to the council's position. Our supplementation philosophy reflects this.

Let's examine more specifically the five reasons why we believe that separate supplements are needed in addition to the balanced and supplement-rich diet we recommended earlier. The biggest flaw in the National Research Council's position that you can get everything you need from a balanced diet is that they overlook the fact that few people actually consistently eat the recommended diet. Poor eating habits start the minute we are weaned from baby food. Even people who do eat several servings of fruits and vegetables in the summer may have a low intake due to limited availability in the winter. We trust that, having taken our nutritional recommendations to heart, you are eating a good diet. But we would be naive indeed to expect that all of you are eating a perfect (or even near-perfect) diet all of the time. Thus, compensating for any such shortcomings is the first good reason for recommending supplements.

The next reason to consider supplements and especially trace minerals, is the variability of nutrients in our food supply. Practically speaking, after numerous seasons of farming on the same soil, trace minerals can be depleted. Since farmers generally refertilize their soil only with nitrogen compounds and the minerals phosphorous and potassium, many of the other minerals you need are simply inadequate in the foods you eat. The plants will not grow well if *all* the trace minerals are gone, but they grow just fine with a smaller trace mineral content than you may need.

It is also true that the more refined, or processed, our food becomes, the less likely it is to contain adequate nutrients. Of course, some refinement is necessary for good health. Some unrefined foods (which is what our shorter-lived ancestors ate) such as unpasteurized milk, can lead to all sorts of problems. It is also true that because processing is known to deplete the nutritional value of foods, the government requires enrichment of certain processed foods with some vitamins. But enrichment with trace minerals is not a requirement and is often not done in the food-manufacturing industry. Thus, we recommend trace mineral supplementation because these ingredients may have been lost in processing.

A natural consequence of aging is a decrease in our ability to digest and absorb many nutrients. This is a well-established fact in geriatric medicine. It is therefore possible to be eating properly but still have some deficiencies if you can't absorb or utilize these nutrients properly. Also, as older folks lose muscle and their metabolism slows, they often eat less. Since their total intake of food is lower, their intake of nutrients such as trace minerals is lower as well—even though they may be needing these nutrients more than ever.

Finally, *treating* disease often requires people to consume nutrients in quantities higher than they get in foods, even with a balanced diet. This is in sharp contrast to eating well enough simply to *prevent* deficiency diseases such as scurvy, pellagra, or beriberi. For example, although the RDA for vitamin E is 10 IU (international units), 100 to 800 IU of vitamin E has been shown in several research studies to be effective for the prevention of heart disease and cataracts and the treatment of Alzheimer's disease. To get the amount of vitamin E you would need to obtain these benefits strictly from food, you would have to consume large quantities of fat and thousands of extra calories daily.

For these reasons, we believe it is important and entirely rational to rely on a good diet for most of the nutrition you need and then to augment that diet with supplements specific to the treatment of your arthritis.

Minerals/Trace Minerals

The minerals calcium, magnesium, silicon, and zinc, and the trace minerals boron, chromium, copper, selenium, and manganese are potentially of great importance both to your general health and to the treatment of your osteoarthritis. Let us now summarize for you the importance of each of these. Research on many of them is continuing rapidly, and therefore we shall try to include both what is proved about these trace minerals and what is suspected and under review.

Boron
This mineral has broad and diverse effects on the human body. It is involved in calcium and bone metabolism and even helps regulate certain hormones, such as testosterone, estrogen, and

calcitonin. Additionally, boron has some antioxidant and anti-inflammatory properties. A number of animal studies and a few small human studies suggest that boron exerts certain indirect effects on mineral and bone metabolism and on osteoarthritis.

We can't say that a lack of boron causes osteoarthritis, or that taking the mineral will cure the disease. However, there seems to be a correlation between osteoarthritis and dietary boron intake. In areas where intake of boron is low, the incidence of osteoarthritis is high. But in regions where people take in more boron, the disease is less frequent and less severe. Also, the boron content of the tissues in the hip joints of normal and osteoarthritic patients has been shown to vary significantly—the normal joints having almost twice the concentration of boron. Finally, at least one experimental pilot study looked at improvement in pain taking boron versus a placebo in ten patients with osteoarthritis.[1] The results of this small study indicated that boron caused a considerable improvement.

We recommend that you take a supplemental dose of 1.5–3 mg of boron daily.

Calcium

There is good documentation that the average person does not get enough calcium in his or her diet. (The recommended amount is between 1,000 to 1,500 mg per day, but the national average consumed is only about 750 mg per day.) While no direct connection between a lack of calcium and *osteoarthritis* has been uncovered through research, there is unanimous agreement that a lack of calcium contributes to *osteoporosis,* a widespread problem, particularly in older women. Besides calcium (and vitamin D) deficiency, osteoporosis is mainly brought on by low levels of the male and female hormones, estrogen and testosterone, and by insufficient weight-bearing exercise. Osteoporosis contributes to an estimated 1.5 million

1. R. L. Travers and G. C. Rennie, "Clinical Trial-Boron and Arthritis," *Townsend Lett.* 83 (1990): 360.

fractures annually and has a huge impact on society. These fractures, especially in the spine, can greatly aggravate the pain and disability caused by osteoarthritis. Therefore, prevention of osteoporosis is important, and making sure you get enough calcium is the key to doing this.

The amount of calcium you need to take supplementarily depends on how much dairy you include in your diet. Calcium citrate is often better tolerated than other types. Avoid oyster-shell, bone meal, and dolomite forms of calcium since they may contain unacceptable amounts of lead and other contaminants. The following table shows you the amount of calcium you need to take daily.

Servings of Dairy Consumed	Amount of Supplemental Calcium Women Need	Amount of Supplemental Calcium Men Need
0	1,200 mg	900 mg
1	900 mg	600 mg
2	600 mg	300 mg
3	300 mg	0 mg

Note: 1 serving of dairy = 8 ounces of milk, 1.5 ounces of cheese, or 6 ounces of yogurt (not frozen yogurt, which is actually low in calcium). Also good to remember is that lowfat (or nonfat) and regular dairy products have the same amount of calcium.

Chromium

Chromium is an essential cofactor for the hormone insulin. Insulin is involved in regulation of the metabolism of carbohydrates, fats, and proteins. Excess insulin production and increased insulin resistance are features of adult-onset diabetes. Chromium supplements in chromium-deficient diabetic individuals can help improve their clinical picture. Though there is a link between diabetes and osteoarthritis, no direct link has been established between chromium *intake* and osteoarthritis. Nevertheless, it is prudent to mitigate a chromium deficiency, if it exists.

We therefore recommend that you take a supplemental dose of 50–200 micrograms (mcg) per day. Patients with adult-onset diabetes may consider taking higher doses, under the recommendation of their physician.

Copper

Copper bracelets have been used for decades as a ''cure'' for arthritis, and the people who wear them swear that they work. But they don't have any real, proven benefit. *Oral* copper supplements, however, may have some benefit in those who are copper deficient. Copper serves as a component of some of the enzymes involved in collagen and bone formation, in antioxidant activities, and in generating ATP (energy) within cells. In addition, copper may have some weak antioxidant properties of its own by helping convert iron (an oxidant) into a less harmful state.

The metabolism of copper is related to the amount of zinc in the body. People who take too much zinc may trigger a copper deficiency, since excess zinc can lead to a reduction in copper levels.

Our recommendation for the proper supplemental dosage of copper is to take 1–2 mg per day.

Magnesium

Magnesium plays a pivotal role in the musculoskeletal system including the bones, muscles, and other soft tissues. Some surveys report that up to 30 percent of some adult populations studied have low levels of magnesium. Supplemental magnesium is often necessary when calcium supplements are taken because the body's absorption and utilization of both are related.

We recommend that you take an amount of magnesium that is one-third of your daily calcium intake. If you take too much magnesium, it may result in loose stools (Milk of Magnesia got its name from the mineral magnesium).

Manganese

Manganese is a component of some of the enzymes responsible for the formation of cartilage, especially proteoglycans and collagen. Deficiencies have long been recognized in the veterinary community as a cause of joint and other musculoskeletal problems in animals. There is some evidence that the human body's ability to utilize manganese declines with age. Thus there is a significant possibility that there may be a connection between the development of osteoarthritis in the elderly and declining manganese levels in aging cartilage.

We recommend a supplemental dosage of manganese, about 10–30 mg per day.

Selenium

Selenium is found in seafood, whole grains, and some nuts. It is one of the components of the four ACES, the major antioxidants, and is discussed in Chapter 6.

Selenium is unique in that not only is it an important trace mineral, but it is also an antioxidant. For that reason, we feel it is important to discuss this unique mineral in this section, and later in the antioxidant discussion.

We recommend a dose of 50–200 mcg per day.

Silicon

Within the last decade, silicon has been recognized as performing an important role in bone and cartilage formation. Silicon's primary effect is in strengthening connective collagen tissues and on the mineralization of bone. Children who were hospitalized and getting their nutrition entirely by artificial intravenous feeding, and who also had low serum levels of silicon, were found to have deficiencies in bone density.[2]

As a result, we believe that it is reasonably safe to suggest the addition of silicon to your diet. It seems highly unlikely

2. A. A. Moukarzel, A. L. Buchman, M. Song, M. E. Ament, "Is Silicon Deficiency an Etiological Factor in Osteopenia of Parenteral Nutrition Bone Disease of Children?" *J. Am. Coll. Nutr.* 11, no. 5 (1992): 601.

that it could do harm, since some people consume large quantities of sand, mostly silicon dioxide, inadvertently left on vegetables and fruits by incomplete washing, and suffer no adverse effects. As with all supplements, in the absence of adequate research, one should be conservative.

Silicon should be ingested through foods known to be beneficial in many other ways as well, or taken in only low dosages as a supplement (less than 5–10 mg per day).

Zinc

Zinc has long been associated with wound healing. It is intimately involved in cartilage metabolism, and serves, with copper, as a vital component to help certain enzymes work properly. Several small, double-blind studies have used zinc supplements in patients with rheumatoid and psoriatic arthritis, but not with osteoarthritis. The majority of these studies showed significant benefits compared to placebo in terms of reduction of joint pain and tenderness.

We recommend a supplemental dosage of 5–10 mg per day of zinc.

A Special Note on Mineral Supplementation

Not everyone who takes mineral supplements experiences a dramatic, or even noticeable, improvement in his or her symptoms of osteoarthritis, at least not right away. Those who do notice a rapid effect are likely to have been deficient in one or more of these minerals. But you must remember, the higher dosages often needed to correct deficiencies should not be used as maintenance doses, since this may lead to toxicity over months or years. All trace minerals if consumed in excess are likely to be bad for you. For this reason, we recommend taking *daily* dosages at the low end of the range recommended by manufacturers. The following table reflects our recommendations:

MINERAL	DAILY DOSAGE
Boron	1.5–3 mg
Calcium	As per chart (page 188)
Chromium	50–200 mcg
Copper	1–2 mg
Magnesium	one-third of calcium intake
Manganese	10–30 mg
Selenium	50–200 mcg
Silicon	5–10 mg
Zinc	5–10 mg

By eating properly and supplementing your diet with these low doses of trace minerals, you'll correct deficiencies, treat your OA, and avoid possible toxicity due to excess or inappropriate intake.

There is also one trace mineral that is widely used, which we do *not* recommend for osteoarthritis sufferers: iron.

Iron is mainly necessary to form hemoglobin, the molecule responsible for carrying oxygen in the blood. Low iron stores can lead to iron-deficiency anemia. With those who suffer from arthritis, we are more concerned with *high* iron stores, especially from the condition called hemochromatosis, the "iron storage disease." Hemochromatosis is an inherited condition that leads to accumulation of excess iron throughout the body. This eventually leads to heart disease, diabetes, and, interestingly, secondary osteoarthritis. Fortunately, hemochromatosis is easily screened by the use of a simple test of the blood's level of iron and ferritin (a storage form of iron in the body).

There is even some evidence that excess iron, even if you don't have hemochromatosis, can cause more oxidation of tissues in the body (remember, we want oxidation limited; that's why we recommend antioxidants). People with excess iron are usually told to limit their intake of iron-containing foods (red meat being the biggest offender) and to donate their blood. Blood donation effectively reduces iron stores as your body draws on these stores to make new blood cells to replace the ones donated. Unless your physician tells you specifically to take supplemental iron, don't take any. And be aware that iron is often included in multivitamin tablets. So choose one without iron. More people have excess amounts of iron after age fifty than are iron deficient.

What About Other Minerals?

There are many other minerals we have not discussed or made recommendations for supplementation. The reason for this is either that people are not generally deficient in these minerals and obtain sufficient (and sometimes even excess amounts) in their diet, or that there is no significant evidence of health benefit from taking them in supplemental or other forms.

Antioxidants

Although we don't yet understand how or why primary osteoarthritis begins, one theory holds that free radicals either trigger or exacerbate damage to the joints by indiscriminately destroying healthy tissue. Free radicals are unbalanced molecules that seek to stabilize themselves by "stealing" electrons from other molecules. The "theft" calms the now-stable free radical but damages the other molecule. The loss of a single molecule is of little concern, but if there are billions of free radicals assaulting the body every day, these tiny "bites" can add up to a great deal of damage over time. Free radical damage is felt to be a major contributing factor to joint damage, heart disease, cancer, and aging. These harmful molecules arise in the body naturally, as by-products of normal metabolism as well as from outside factors such as pollution.

The Four ACES

The four most important antioxidants are vitamins A, C, and E and the mineral selenium (the four ACES). We cannot emphasize enough that making sure your body gets enough of these nutrients is vital to your overall health, as well as to treating your osteoarthritis. Generally, we feel that it is better to ingest these supplements in your normal food than by taking pills, but you should consider adding low dosages of supplements to your daily routine. With vitamins C and E, at least, the amounts of the antioxidants you'll need are higher than you'd get in your average diet. Always remember, however, that just because some is good does not mean more is better! Megadoses of any nutrient can have adverse health effects.

The specific daily doses we recommend (to fight arthritis and maintain good health) are:

vitamin A	5,000 IU
vitamin C	500–4,000 mg
vitamin E	100–400 IU
selenium	50–200 mcg

Vitamin "P"

Several other antioxidants can work with the four ACES to keep joints healthy. The bioflavonoids—quercetin, hesperidin, rutin, the catechins, and more—also have antioxidant properties. Originally called "vitamin P," this group of 200–plus plant chemicals helps to control free radicals, improve collagen's ability to form a strong matrix, prevent collagen destruction caused by inflammation, and speed wound healing. These phytochemicals also help to strengthen the tiny blood vessels called capillaries and are useful in treating bleeding gums. We recommend that you add bioflavonoids, also known simply as flavonoids, to your diet. They are often included in vitamin C tablets and with antioxidant supplements. The recommended amount is 250–1000 mg of mixed or citrus bioflavonoids twice a day.

The B Vitamins

The B vitamins, often called the B-complex vitamins, consist of B_1 (thiamine), B_2 (riboflavin), B_3 (niacin), B_6 (pyridoxine), and B_{12} (cyanocobalamin). Folic acid, pantothenic acid, and biotin are other vitamins usually included in the B-complex family. Much new evidence has implicated deficiencies of certain B vitamins and folic acid in several conditions, including heart disease (probably due to the high levels of homocysteine in the blood with B deficiencies) and neural tube defects. Vitamin B deficiencies are also well-known causes of certain neurological conditions, including dementia, and a type of anemia of the blood. Interestingly, people deficient in B-complex vitamins also have low SAMe levels. (SAMe is discussed in detail later in this chapter.) Correcting these deficiencies can normalize SAMe levels. This makes sense, since B vitamins are intimately involved in the enzymes responsible for SAMe production in the body.

We recommend the RDAs for the B-complex vitamins. Fortunately, most multivitamin tablets contain the recommended amounts. An added benefit of taking a multivitamin is that you should get our recommended doses of vitamin A and D in most multivitamin formulas. You need to take additional C and E, along with the trace minerals, but taking a multivitamin can help to decrease the number of tablets or capsules you need to ingest in a day.

Vitamin D

Vitamin D may also be a helpful nutrient in the fight against arthritis. We've known for a long time that a lack of vitamin D can cause rickets and other bone problems. According to a 1996 study published in the *Annals of Internal Medicine,* lack of the vitamin may also speed the progression of osteoarthritis.[3]

Sometimes called the "sunshine vitamin," vitamin D can be made by the body when it's exposed to sunlight. It also comes from food, with our best source being fortified milk. A study involving more than five hundred elderly persons suffering from osteoarthritis of the knee found that those who had the lowest blood levels and intake of the vitamin were three times more likely to see their disease progress, compared to those with the highest levels of the vitamin. The progression of arthritis was verified with X rays taken at the beginning of the study and four years later.

Although we don't know exactly how vitamin D may slow the progression of osteoarthritis, it seems prudent for people with low dietary intakes to take a multivitamin containing 200–400 IU of the vitamin. (The recommended daily allowance for vitamin D is 200 IU.) Until confirmatory studies on vitamin D and osteoarthritis are performed, there appears to be no harm from taking this dose. Too much D can be toxic, however, so keep in mind that the total includes "D" foods and any supplements you are taking.

The Basic Supplement Program

Let us summarize what we recommend. It is actually quite simple, and we urge you to add this basic program of supplements to your intake of chondroitin and glucosamine. It will maximize the effectiveness of your cure, and can be supplied by four small tablets or capsules.

- A multivitamin without iron, but that contains sufficient A, B-complex, and D
- A multimineral that contains all of the recommended minerals
- Vitamin C with bioflavonoids twice per day
- Vitamin E–mixed tocopherols/with mixed carotenoids

3. *Ann Intern Med* 125 (1996): 353–59.

This combination will work effectively to combat your osteoarthritis. It will also improve your overall health. If you have any questions about any supplements, consult your physician or registered dietitian.

Recent Breakthroughs That Could Enhance the Cure: SAMe and Hydrolized Collagen

There are two new breakthroughs that seem to offer considerable potential for the future. The first is a compound called S-Adenosylmethionine, or SAMe for short (pronounced "sammy"). The other is hydrolyzed collagen, which is widely used in Europe and is being launched in this country with a great deal of fanfare.

SAMe

S-Adenosylmethionine may be helpful to arthritis sufferers because of its possible protective effects on cartilage.[4]

SAMe, currently being produced in Europe primarily to treat liver problems and depression, isn't yet available in the United States but is expected within a year. Given its current limited production, it is too expensive for general use in osteoarthritis. (In Europe, at the full treatment dose for osteoarthritis, the cost of SAMe is approximately $15 per day). SAMe is a very sensitive compound. It can be inactivated by heat, light, or moisture. Therefore, it has to be stabilized, coated, and stored in blister packs. It does not keep as a powder or in an uncoated tablet. Nonetheless, these problems can be overcome, and we are anticipating that, as more professionals become aware of its benefits in treating osteoarthritis, SAMe will become readily available at an affordable price.

One word of warning: Several products on the market claim to contain SAMe, but they do not. Sometimes companies try to pass off the amino acid methionine as SAMe, but methionine by itself does not have any effect on arthritis, so it is not

4. *American Journal of Medicine* 83, suppl. 5A (November 20, 1987): 1–4.

a valid substitute. Several researchers have postulated that because SAMe is a "methyl donor" (it donates part of itself to other molecules), other methyl donors could replace SAMe, or at least augment its activity in the body. Betaine (or trimethylglycine, TMG) is one of those compounds. Betaine has actually been shown to increase levels of SAMe in animals and humans. The big question is, Does this translate into the same clinical effect as taking SAMe itself? We'll see as more research is reported. This is an important question, since vitamin marketers will likely start to sell "SAMe complexes," which may contain small amounts of the real, expensive SAMe along with other methyl donors like betaine.

Recent information suggests that SAMe may indeed become a significant addition to the arthritis cure. So let us continue by discussing it in some detail.

How Does SAMe work?

SAMe works in a number of ways to add to the effectiveness of glucosamine and chondroitin. Its main functions seem to be:

- To help produce and stabilize proteoglycans (the water-loving molecules that make up about 15 percent of cartilage). SAMe does this by donating part of itself (a *methyl* group), which helps initiate the process of sulfuration (a necessary step in forming proteoglycans).
- As a precursor of *polyamines*. Polyamines are involved with cell proliferation and protein synthesis, both necessary for newly formed cartilage. Polyamines also possess anti-inflammatory and analgesic properties (so that SAMe may have a direct effect on pain).
- To metabolize itself first to homocysteine and then to cysteine and glutathione. Cysteine and glutathione—as well as the polyamines—are scavengers of free radicals and may well exert effective antioxidant protection to cartilage.

These complicated actions, all working together, may have the effect of protecting the cartilage from attack by certain enzymes, thus allowing the "building" effects of glucosamine and chondroitin to be more effective. In laboratory studies, SAMe has been shown to increase proteoglycan synthesis by the chondrocytes. The studies also support the hypothesis that SAMe may counter the enzymatic attacks on cartilage that are part of the underlying process of osteoarthritis while at the same time stimulating cartilage growth. That is indeed exciting. SAMe has all of the ingredients to be a perfect complement to glucosamine and chondroitin.

At least six double-blind, controlled human trials have been published on the use of SAMe for the treatment of osteoarthritis. These studies have shown that SAMe is effective in reducing osteoarthritis pain and inflammation, not only when compared to a placebo but to standard NSAIDs as well. For instance, a study of eighty-one osteoarthritis patients conducted at the University of Indiana showed that the SAMe treatment group had significantly greater reduction in overall pain than the placebo control group.[5] Moreover, as just stated, clinical studies have indicated that SAMe is as effective as NSAIDs in reducing osteoarthritis pain and inflammation. Such was the result of a double-blind study conducted in Germany, in which thirty-six patients with osteoarthritis were treated either with SAMe or ibuprofen. The pain improvement for the two groups was the same.[6]

But SAMe has two additional benefits over NSAIDs. The first is that SAMe does not have the gastrointestinal side effects associated with NSAIDs. Second, studies have shown that an added benefit of SAMe is that it alleviates depression. As you may recall, depression is a common problem in those with chronic conditions such as osteoarthritis. The evidence for SAMe being an effective antidepressant is based on more than a dozen separate controlled studies conducted at multiple sites, including the Università Cattolica Sacro Cuore School of Medicine in Rome, the University of California at Irvine

5. *Journal of Rheumatology* 21, no. 5 (May 1994): 905–11.
6. *American Journal of Medicine* 83, no. 5A (November 30, 1987): 81–83.

Medical Center, Massachusetts General Hospital, and Harvard Medical School.[7]

Shedding further light on the promising nature of SAMe is the fact that studies on it date back to 1966. Some of these studies have been substantial. For example, in Milan, Italy, a double-blind study involving 734 subjects with osteoarthritis of the knees, hips, spine and/or hands was performed in the mid 1980s. Thirty-three orthopedic and rheumatology centers participated in the study. The study subjects were randomized into three groups: placebo, SAMe, and naproxen (an anti-inflammatory). Though the subjects were treated only for a month, both the naproxen and SAMe groups had significantly less pain and performed better on functional tests than the placebo group. The SAMe group, however, had the best tolerability of the treatment as indicated by the lowest number of side effects and by both the patients' and physicians' judgments.

What about safety? The results of the first long-term trial have been quite impressive. A two-year clinical trial with SAMe was undertaken on 108 patients with osteoarthritis of the knee, hip, and/or spine. The patients received 600 mg of SAMe daily for two weeks, and 400 mg daily until the end of the twenty-fourth month. The clinical symptom severity (morning stiffness, pain at rest or on movement) was assessed weekly for two weeks and then monthly. Improvement of the clinical symptoms occurred within two weeks and continued until the end of the study. Nonspecific side effects occurred in twenty patients, but no one had to stop treatment because of these mild effects. Indeed, no adverse effects were recorded in the last six months of treatment. Detailed laboratory tests were performed at baseline and every six months, and no specific health problems were uncovered. As a side benefit, the authors reported that SAMe supplementation also improved the feelings of depression often associated with osteoarthritis.[8]

7. Reports of these studies were published in *Acta Neurologica Scandinavia. Supplementum* 154 (1994): 7–18; and *Journal of Psychiatric Research* 24, no. 2 (1990): 177–94.

8. *Journal of Medicine* 83, no. 5A (November 20, 1987): 89–94.

The most exciting research related to SAMe involves its potential to have *disease-modifying* effects, as do glucosamine and chondroitin. Does SAMe actually help heal cartilage? Researchers in Berlin performed a prospective study (people were placed in the study, then treated and their progress then followed) of twenty-one patients with osteoarthritis of the finger joints. The researchers used an MRI scanner to evaluate the cartilage in these joints. Two-thirds of the study subjects were given SAMe for three months, one-third were left untreated. Since the patients were not "reporting" their own condition, a placebo was not necessary. The researchers noted a stronger signal emanating from the cartilage on the MRI scans of the treated group. They interpreted this as an actual *structural* improvement compared to the untreated group.[9]

Glucosamine and chondroitin remain the first-line supplements for osteoarthritis. More than 90 percent of the people I have treated respond to a combination of these supplements, assuming that the products they are taking are pure and that they follow the rest of the arthritis cure program. Until the time comes when SAMe, glucosamine, and chondroitin have been studied together, SAMe should be considered only by those (in the minority) who have not had a sufficient response to glucosamine and chondroitin alone.

As with glucosamine and chondroitin supplements, SAMe supplements may take a few weeks before you feel a positive effect. In addition, as with all supplements, we recommend that people take the minimum effective dose. Start with 400–600 mg per day, and consider gradually tapering the dose down over a period of weeks to months to reach the desired effect. SAMe should be taken for at least two months to see if there's an effect.

9. H. Konig, H. Stahl, J. Sieper, and K. J. Wolf, "Magnetic Resonance Tomography of Finger Polyarthritis: Morphology and Cartilage Signals After Ademetionine Therapy" [in German], *Aktuelle Radiologie* 5, no. 1 (January 1995): 36–40.

Hydrolyzed Collagen

Three different products—type II collagen, hydrolyzed collagen, and gelatin—are sometimes confused in popular medical literature, but they are all quite different. Recently, hydrolyzed collagen has been increasingly promoted as a cure for various forms of arthritis. As happens sometimes, the hype is outrunning the truth, since much is still unknown about this product. Clearly, though, there is some fire underneath all the smoke. So let's see if we can clarify what is known and what isn't about the three. First, what are these products and what are the health claims being made for each?

Gelatin is well known and sold under many brand names and, of course, in a variety of desserts and candies. In many countries, notably Germany, it is "known" to have wide-ranging health benefits. However, although it is often referred to as "gelatin," what these countries are referring to when labeling a product gelatin is actually *hydrolyzed collagen.* Gelatin in the form in which we in the United States are all familiar has little or no known beneficial effect on arthritis. Hydrolyzed collagen, a more easily assimilated derivative of gelatin, may be a different matter entirely.

Type II collagen and *hydrolyzed collagen* are two very different types of collagen products, but both are being studied as "chondro-protective" treatments for arthritis. The hypothesis is that they both inhibit cartilage breakdown, improve the supply of nutrients to cartilage tissue, stimulate constructive processes, and thus finally reduce the progress of joint debilitation. However, type II collagen seems to show special promise for reducing the inflammation associated with rheumatoid arthritis. We therefore cover it more thoroughly in Chapter 8.

Ordinary collagen makes up about 15 percent of cartilage. Hydrolyzed collagen, manufactured from the collagenous tissues of animals (such as cow hides and bones), contains large amounts of the amino acids that are found in ordinary collagens. It is these amino acids that help make new collagen, so the theory is that more amino acids should make more collagen and hence more cartilage. The catch is that the amino acids abundant in hydrolyzed collagen are not exactly the same as the ones that become incorporated in new collagen within cartilage.

The FDA has given hydrolyzed collagen a GRAS (Generally Regarded as Safe) rating when sold as a food (as opposed to a drug) product. But recently there has been a strong movement toward marketing hydrolyzed collagen in this country as a chondro-protective treatment for many forms of arthritis, including OA and RA. This follows its widespread use in Europe, where it is routinely recommended by doctors for their arthritic patients. In the light of all this buzz, it is fair to ask if it indeed works.

There have not been any double-blind, placebo-controlled trials on hydrolyzed collagen published in peer review journals. There have been, however, at least two studies conducted in well-established German research institutions but published only in popular, not professional, journals. These articles describe placebo-controlled studies that imply that hydrolyzed collagen has considerable and meaningful efficacy. Unfortunately, since these studies have not been subjected to professional scrutiny, we can place only limited confidence in them. All the preliminary and anecdotal evidence does suggest to us that there is a real possibility that hydrolyzed collagen may have important benefits. The early evidence shows promise, and we are eagerly awaiting the results of research currently underway. Certainly, this product deserves further study.

Considering how many people are taking hydrolyzed collagen—and swearing by it—it is a relief to be able to report that it appears to be well tolerated. The only known side effects are occasional and minor gastrointestinal discomfort such as some bloating, gas, and stomach upset.

Hydrolyzed collagen is usually made in powdered form and mixed into a large glass of water or juice. Dosages range from 5 to 12 grams per day. Two to three months is a sufficient timeframe to know if it is working on your achy joints.

A New Generation of Prescription NSAIDs

A new generation of prescription NSAIDs, called COX-II inhibitors, promise to eliminate many of the side effects seen with ibuprofen, naproxen, aspirin, and other NSAIDs.[10]

Many physicians are eagerly looking forward to the arrival of the COX-II inhibitors, for NSAID-induced side effects are a serious problem. More than seventy million prescriptions for NSAIDs are filled every year in the United States, and many more people purchase over-the-counter ibuprofen, aspirin, and other NSAIDs. The resulting gastrointestinal and other side effects can be serious—and quite costly.

We don't fully understand how the NSAIDs block pain and reduce inflammation, but it's felt that they do so by suppressing an enzyme called cyclooxygenase (COX). Specifically, they interfere with two types of COX, type I and II. COX-I protects the stomach, intestines, and kidneys by helping to produce certain prostaglandins (chemical substances involved in regulating various physiologic processes in certain tissues). We want to have plenty of this "good" COX. COX-II produces the prostaglandins that can cause inflammation and pain. As far as arthritis is concerned, this is the "bad" COX.

The NSAIDs help arthritis sufferers by preventing the "bad" COX-II from producing the pain-inducing prostaglandins. But they also stop the "good" COX-I from guarding the stomach and intestines. That makes the NSAIDs a two-edged sword: They help by reducing the pain-causing prostaglandins, but they hurt by reducing the body's ability to protect the stomach and intestines. Unprotected, the stomach and intestines are easy targets for ulcers and other problems.

The new COX-II inhibitors seem to get around this problem by interfering mostly with the production of "bad" COX-II, leaving the "good" COX-I alone. If they work as well as the early studies promise, they will represent a major step forward

10. D. Y. Graham, "Nonsteroidal Anti-inflammatory Drugs, Helicobacter Pylori, and Ulcers: Where We Stand," *Am J Gastroenterology* 91, no. 10 (July 1997): 2080–86.

in the treatment of the pain of arthritis and other musculo-skeletal problems.

But remember COX-II inhibitors do not cure arthritis. They may relieve pain and inflammation, and they may do so with fewer side effects, but they do nothing about solving the underlying problem.

Some doctors are suggesting that we set aside glucosamine and chondroitin sulfates because the COX-II inhibitors will be out soon. But although they are an improvement over the old NSAIDs, again, they do not cure osteoarthritis. So if your doctor suggests that you try a COX-II inhibitor for your osteoarthritis, ask him or her whether the medicine will really solve the problem—or if you'll have to remain on the COX-II inhibitor, or some other medicine, for the rest of your life. Then ask about glucosamine and chondroitin sulfates.

8

Rheumatoid Arthritis: New Hope for Sufferers

Rheumatoid arthritis is a very different disease from osteoarthritis. So different, in fact, that it's a shame that they share *arthritis* in their names, for this just seems to confuse people. Whereas osteoarthritis is the wearing down of the cartilage, a problem that can be dramatically improved by the arthritis cure, rheumatoid arthritis involves the destruction of the joints by an *immune* mechanism—the body literally attacks the joints as though they were foreign invaders. There are about 2.5 million people with rheumatoid arthritis in the United States, less than one-tenth the number of those with osteoarthritis. Compared to the (generally) slow course of osteoarthritis, joint destruction in rheumatoid arthritis can occur rapidly. In a few months or years, a victim of rheumatoid arthritis may suffer with painful, deformed joints that have limited function and may even need replacing. To make matters worse, unlike osteoarthritis, rheumatoid arthritis often affects areas of the body besides the joints and can leave its sufferers with fatigue and fevers, along with skin, lung, blood vessel, and even heart problems.

Though a variety of standard medical treatments are available for sufferers of rheumatoid arthritis, many patients have difficulty tolerating these treatments and are on the constant lookout for something better, something less likely to cause harmful side effects. These patients are looking for *alternatives* to standard therapy. Others are getting fair to good results with their standard therapies and simply are looking for substances that will augment their treatment program. This is the hallmark of *complementary* treatments.

There now is some new hope. New treatments can augment, and even replace, some standard medical therapies for rheumatoid arthritis. The most exciting new treatment is *oral enzyme therapy*. But don't count out glucosamine and chondroitin, type II collagen, or the anti-inflammatory oils and the soon-to-be-released prescription medications COX-II inhibitors and TNF antagonists (genetically engineered molecules that block the substances that lead to pain and inflammation) for rheumatoid arthritis. Finally, the prescription drugs minocycline and the new antimetabolite Arava (leflunomide), show promise in preventing and reversing joint damage in rheumatoid arthritis.

A Note of Common Sense
Most cases of *osteoarthritis* are handled by family physicians, internists, sports medicine physicians, or orthopedic surgeons. *Rheumatoid arthritis* patients, in contrast, are usually managed with the help of a *rheumatologist,* a medical specialist who focuses on treating the hundred or so various forms of arthritis.

Since there are proven treatments known to improve the course of rheumatoid arthritis, please be sure to consult with your physician regarding the use of any alternative or complementary treatments. Do not blindly abandon the known, standard therapies for alternative ones, since this could result in a flare-up of your rheumatoid arthritis and cause significant harm. On the other hand, if your doctor balks at the idea of using nonstandard treatments, please ask if he or she is familiar with the available medical literature related to these treatments. It is okay if a doctor doesn't know, but no professional should say a treatment is no good if he or she has not mastered the relevant information. Remember, every single treatment in medical history was nonstandard at one point! Also, physicians read less than one-tenth of 1 percent of the available biomedical literature. There's a lot of good science that takes years or even decades to become mainstream in the medical field. Our work in this book, and in *The Arthritis Cure,* is intended to accelerate the progress of incorporating good science into the field of arthritis.

Oral Enzyme Therapy

A Primer on Enzymes

It is often difficult to grasp that the body is really a collection of cells and the substances made by those cells. The seventy-five *trillion* cells in the body are constantly creating, destroying, and altering various molecules in a variety of chemical reactions. The term for these chemical reactions in the body is *metabolism.* Metabolism, or metabolic activity, is the hallmark of living tissue. A *catalyst* allows chemical reactions to proceed easier by using less energy, much like the wheels on the bottom of a piece of luggage allow you to walk through an airport more easily than if you had to lift and carry it. There is a special term for catalysts in living cells—*enzymes.* More than three thousand different enzymes have been identified in the human body. Each enzyme has a specific job by serving as a catalyst for one particular chemical reaction. Enzymes are basically protein in composition, and many require certain minerals to function (we discuss the importance of minerals in more detail in Chapter 7). If you ever wondered what certain vitamins and minerals actually do in the body, the answer is in their intimate relationship with enzymes. For instance, almost all minerals are known to be part of one or more enzymes. Indeed, all mineral-containing enzymes become nonfunctional without their mineral constituents.

Enzymes have a wide range of functions. There are enzymes that allow us to break down starches, such as bread, into simple sugar molecules; enzymes that incorporate glucosamine into chains that form proteoglycans in cartilage; and enzymes that cause the body to produce certain chemicals, called cytokines, which can result in inflammation and pain. You may not have been aware of it, but you have been eating enzymes your entire life. Not only are they contained within all vegetables, fruits, grains, and animal products, enzymes are added into many processed foods as well, to "age" certain foods such as cheese and wine, and to enhance flavor. The next time you look at a food label, check to see if the word *enzymes* appears in the list of ingredients.

Enzymes are usually classified into different groups, depending on the general functions they perform. Most of the time, a specific enzyme has the suffix *-ase* in its name. For instance, amylase, protease, and lipase are categories of enzymes that are involved with the breakdown of sugars, proteins, and fats, respectively.

Though the initial discovery of enzymes occurred about two hundred years ago, scientists are still learning more about the enzymes responsible for the manifestations of disease. More than fifteen years ago, scientists learned that the enzyme HMG-CoA reductase (they often have long, fancy names) was responsible for how much cholesterol people make in their livers (and hence is dumped into the blood). A drug was developed to block this enzyme; now there are five drugs on the market that do this, and the blood of people taking these drugs has proved to have lower cholesterol levels as a result. Even better, these drugs have been shown to be *disease-modifying* agents for blocked arteries (atherosclerosis). People with high cholesterol taking these drugs have a lower chance of having a heart attack than those with high cholesterol who are not taking the drugs. Much of the pharmaceutical industry has been focused on finding enzyme *blockers,* drugs that in some manner block the action of a specific enzyme. But there are other ways of treating or preventing diseases—by *increasing* the level of certain "good" enzymes. Good is in quotes because, enzymes are really neither good nor bad. Disease often occurs when one enzyme system is out of proportion to another. In osteoarthritis, for instance, when the catabolic (dissolving) enzyme activity overshadows the anabolic (building-up) enzymes, the cartilage slowly degrades over time, leading to pain, changes in the underlying bone, etc.

Glucosamine and chondroitin help to rebalance the enzyme systems back toward normal. That's why they are such a huge advantage over the NSAIDs, which simply block the enzyme cyclooxygenase without addressing the consequences of the subsequent enzyme imbalance.

More than thirty years ago, scientists began to unravel the enzymes responsible for the complex phenomenon called *inflammation,* which is believed to be at the heart of certain diseases, including rheumatoid arthritis. Excess inflammation leads to unnecessary tissue destruction and pain. The inflammatory reaction in the body is actually quite common, not just limited to autoimmune diseases. Almost all acute injuries, for instance, involve inflammation. The inflammatory process involves hundreds of different chemicals, hormones, and cells, and is extremely complicated. Though some inflammation is good, in certain conditions or diseases, such as a severe ankle sprain or rheumatoid arthritis, the body may overreact, causing more harm than good. In these cases we need to control the inflammation so it does not get out of hand. One of the best ways is by manipulation of the enzymes involved in the inflammatory process. Only a fraction of the three thousand enzymes are actually involved in the inflammatory process. Though we still have much to learn, there are certain enzyme combinations that, when taken orally, can reduce the inflammatory reaction before it leads to damage.

Enzyme preparations

Dozens of clinical studies on various enzymes (used for more than a dozen inflammation-related diseases) have been performed and published over the past four decades. Studies on oral enzyme supplementation in arthritis are even currently underway in the United States, as the American medical community begins to see the light on the promise of these agents. In Germany, the ninth best selling pharmaceutical agent (out of 2,800 products) is a mixture of enzymes used to reduce inflammation. Enzyme preparations have been shown to be at least as effective as anti-inflammatory drugs, such as NSAIDs, in treating many different conditions, including arthritis. The incidence of side effects with the enzymes is very low, a drastic difference to the NSAIDs. These preparations are available without a prescription, as they are sold as nutritional supplements. The FDA recognizes them as GRAS (Generally Recognized As Safe) since they are mostly derived from food products, with little or no modification other than purification.

The enzyme combinations that have anti-inflammatory effects and have undergone extensive study usually involve combinations of bromelain and trypsin, though many often contain papain, chymotrypsin, and occasionally other enzymes. Rutin—a bioflavonoid, not technically an enzyme—possesses direct anti-inflammatory action and is usually included in these mixtures. Let's familiarize ourselves with each of these components.

BROMELAIN

Extracted from the stem of ripe pineapples, bromelain mainly helps to reduce swelling and breaks up some of the antigen-antibody complexes involved in autoimmune reactions. Antigen-antibody complexes are normally broken down by certain cells in the body called *macrophages*. The accumulation of these complexes in tissues is believed to be one of the major causes of tissue destruction in autoimmune diseases like rheumatoid arthritis. Bromelain has lesser but still important activities, such as changing the receptors on cells (where signal chemicals attach and cause inflammation) and directly decreasing cellular activity (in the cells responsible for inflammation). Bromelain is inactivated at levels of acidity less than pH3 (the acid in the stomach is pH2, which is ten times more acidic than pH3). To prevent breakdown in the stomach before being absorbed in the small intestine, oral bromelain supplements have a special coating.

TRYPSIN AND CHYMOTRYPSIN

Both are digestive enzymes found in most animals, including humans, and both are extracted from the pancreas of pigs. Their role as anti-inflammatory agents is to help break down small clots of the material *fibrin*, break up antigen-antibody complexes, and alter the receptors on cells involved with inflammation.

PAPAIN

Extracted from the unripe fruit of the papaya tree, this enzyme is the strongest in the group in breaking up the antigen-antibody complexes involved in autoimmune reactions. Like bromelain, papain is inactivated in overly acidic environments (like the stomach) and must have a special enteric coating to prevent it from being broken down and inactivated.

RUTIN

This bioflavonoid has strong anti-inflammatory effects in the body. Its mechanism of action differs from the NSAIDs, and it does not have any of the serious side effects of the NSAIDs. It is usually taken in the form of Rutosid•$3H_2O$.

Studies Involving Oral Enzymes and Arthritis

The best news about oral enzymes is their long history of use and the quality of clinical data gathered. Oral enzyme mixtures have been studied head to head with NSAIDs, placebos, and even gold. Gold is a standard, disease-modifying treatment for some with RA, but it can lead to significant side effects, such as liver problems and disorders of the blood.

In patients with moderate or severe cases of rheumatoid arthritis, *immunosuppressive* drugs such as methotrexate and cyclosporin are used to control inflammation. Methotrexate was first used in chemotherapy for cancer. It has become the drug of choice for severe rheumatoid arthritis because of disease-modifying (joint tissue improvement) capability. Its use does not come without risk, however. Methotrexate can lead to osteoporosis, liver damage, and certain blood disorders. Fortunately, the simultaneous use of anti-inflammatory enzyme mixtures allows some patients to be able to decrease their dose of methotrexate and (it is hoped) avoid its potentially serious side effects.

How Are Enzymes Taken?
Orally, usually in specially coated tablets or capsules, two to three times per day, thirty to forty minutes before meals. Enzymes are better absorbed on an empty stomach. Some enzyme preparations are delivered intravenously and even as retention enemas. Oral delivery is the preferred route for arthritis sufferers.

What Doses Are Recommended?
The following table describes the (approximate) desired dose for the various oral enzymes. The starting dose is what you take the first week or two of therapy, before cutting down to the maintenance dose. You can gradually cut down the maintenance dose once you notice a prolonged improvement or remission. Some people stay on enzyme therapy for many years, while others need them for just a few weeks or months. Remember, the daily dose is usually split into two to three doses, each taken (preferably) thirty to forty minutes before meals, or not less than sixty minutes after a meal.

Enzyme	Starting Daily Dose (mg/day)	Daily Maintenance Dose (mg/day)	Minimal Enzyme Activity per milligram (in FIP units)
Bromelain	650	450	4.5
Trypsin	350	250	13.5
Chymotrypsin	15	10	270
Papain	900	600	1.3
Rutin*	750	500	NA

*Rutin is not technically an enzyme.

Pancreatin, a mixture of the enzymes of the pancreatic juices, is extracted from animals, and may also be used in some preparations. The recommended dosage is 1000–1500 mg/day (minimum of 3 FIP units for proteolytic activity).

Though the milligram dose is important, equally important is the potency or activity of each of these enzymes. Enzyme activity measures how well the enzyme does its job. I liken this to the octane value for the gasoline for your car. Most cars need gas that has an octane activity or value of at least eighty-seven. Some sporty cars can only use gas which is above ninety-one octane. If you tried to use gas with an octane rating of sixty, your car would not run. Similarly, if you take an enzyme product with an enzyme activity that is too low, the enzyme will not do its job, and you'll be wasting your time and money. There is an international standard for measuring enzyme activity. The standard unit of measure is the FIP, which stands for the Fédération Internationale Pharmaceutique. (Actually, the activity of supplements is nothing new and is not limited to enzymes. Vitamin A is typically measured in *retinol* units, Vitamin E in IU, or *international* units.)

What Should I Expect and When?

Substances (like NSAIDs) that block enzymes are usually quick acting. Since oral enzyme supplements work by altering certain cellular mechanisms, the beneficial effect may not be noticed for at least a week (sometimes even up to a couple of months). Interestingly, this is about the same time frame for glucosamine and chondroitin to demonstrate their effects. One difference between the enzymes and glucosamine and chondroitin, however, is that patients may feel *worse* for three to seven days after starting the enzymes. This is important to note. If you are taking NSAIDs, do not try and wean off of them for a week or two after starting the enzymes (and there's no problem taking the two simultaneously). You'll soon note that there may be no need for the NSAIDs. The enzymes will eventually decrease pain and often improve certain laboratory values related to your rheumatoid arthritis, as your doctor will note as he or she follows your blood tests during routine office visits.

Side Effects, Contraindications, and Drug Interactions of Oral Enzymes

The most common side effect reported is a harmless change in the consistency, color, or odor of stools. High doses taken all at once (instead of split into three doses per day) can lead to a sense of fullness or gas in the abdomen. Anything taken by mouth can lead to allergic reactions, but the incidence of allergy with oral enzymes is exceedingly low. The major contraindications are for those who have problems with bleeding, such as those with severe liver disease or hemophilia (or other inherited or acquired clotting disorders) and dialysis patients. The enzymes can prolong clotting times, so these patients should be monitored closely if enzymes are to be used. No significant drug interactions have been reported, besides an increase in the concentration of certain antibiotics when they are taken simultaneously with oral enzymes. Overall, oral enzymes are among the best-tolerated supplements on the market.

Can Oral Enzymes Be Taken with Glucosamine and Chondroitin?

Yes. There is no known interaction between these supplements. In fact, for those with signs of inflammation (redness, warmth, swelling, and pain), oral anti-inflammatory enzymes are an excellent partner to glucosamine and chondroitin.

What to Watch out for When Choosing a Brand of Enzyme Supplements

Some companies sell enzymes without special coatings or delivery mechanisms to prevent breakdown (and deactivation) in the stomach. In this case, the enzymes may help with digestion but will not enter the bloodstream or exert the desired anti-inflammatory effect. Just because a product appears to have the correct quantities of enzymes on the label does not mean that you will be able to absorb these enzymes. Before picking a particular brand, try to find out if the company has evidence to support that the product actually gets absorbed in the body.

The Impact of Chondroitin and Glucosamine on Rheumatoid Arthritis

Since *The Arthritis Cure* was published in January 1997, people with rheumatoid arthritis have wondered whether they should follow the program. *The Arthritis Cure* treatment program was developed for osteoarthritis, but there is early research evidence that the combination of glucosamine and chondroitin may actually help in the alleviation of rheumatoid arthritis symptoms as well. Appendix A details a study using the combination of these supplements to *prevent* the onset of experimentally induced rheumatoid arthritis in animals. The best news: The case reports of success in people using these supplements for rheumatoid arthritis keep piling in. We hope that this will stimulate some research interest to study and verify these anecdotal reports. Nevertheless (subject to your doctor's agreement, of course), we do encourage patients with rheumatoid arthritis to follow the entire *Arthritis Cure* treatment program, including glucosamine and chondroitin—plus the other *maximizing* steps presented in this book—for two reasons.

Sometimes, patients with rheumatoid arthritis are also suffering from osteoarthritis. *The Arthritis Cure,* in dealing with the latter, greatly eases the discomfort of the sufferer. It is bad enough that joints with worn cartilage from osteoarthritis grind and ache; it is that much worse if they are also inflamed and swollen. Glucosamine and chondroitin do help with inflammation and, by allowing the eroded cartilage to heal, can only help the overall situation.

The other components of *The Arthritis Cure* and *Maximizing the Arthritis Cure* have unquestionable benefit in those with most forms of arthritis. These interventions—the exercise, diet, and behavioral components—are now well known and accepted and have become standards in traditional therapy for rheumatoid arthritis.

Anti-Inflammatory Fatty Acids

The normal palliative treatment for rheumatoid arthritis is the use of NSAIDs for their pain relief and anti-inflammatory action, especially in mild cases. But of course these have side effects. Fortunately, however, there are now a number of alternative approaches that provide significant anti-inflammatory effects with few if any side effects. Patients using these oils typically report less morning stiffness, joint pain, and swelling. Let's summarize the anti-inflammatory fatty acids, or oils, here.

- *Gamma-linolenic acid (GLA)* is a precursor of the "good" prostaglandins that reduce inflammation, improve blood flow, and prevent platelets from sticking together unnecessarily. You'll find GLA in borage seed oil, black currant seed, and primrose oil, in order of decreasing amounts. A minimum dose of 1.4 grams of GLA per day for as long as three months appears to be necessary for full response. A few small, placebo-controlled studies using GLA supplements have been published in the mainstream rheumatology literature.[1]

You should be getting all you need of these two anti-inflammatories if you are eating a healthful diet with plenty of vegetables and fish. However, if inflammation is a real problem for you, you can add them as supplements. But be wary, because occasionally they can worsen, rather than relieve, inflammation in the first few days of use. So use them cautiously, starting off with small amounts to see how you react.

• *Eicosapentaenoic acid (EPA),* an omega-3 fatty acid found in fish and marine plants and flax seeds, helps block inflammation. In a reasonably well-balanced diet, you should be getting enough EPA. However, if you suffer from severely inflamed joints, you may want to increase the amount. The recommended amount is 2.6 grams of EPA per day for the full effect. You can do that eating more fish, or by consuming flax seeds or flax oil, the latter usually available as a supplement.

Flaxseed oil is the preferred source of omega-3 fatty acids, since about 50 percent of it is omega-3. Note, the oil must be fresh, cold-pressed, and can be stored in the freezer, if it's not going to be used, for a couple of days. Do not use it for cooking. Supplements of omega-3 fatty acids have been shown to help in those with rheumatoid arthritis. In a twelve-month double-blind, controlled study, ninety patients received daily supplements of either 2.6 grams of omega-3 fatty acids, 6 grams of olive oil, or 1.3 grams of omega-3 fatty acids plus 3 grams of olive (the olive oil was meant to be a placebo). The patients taking the 2.6 grams of omega-3 fatty acids per day

1. D. Rothman, et al., "Botanical Lipids: Effects on Inflammation, Immune Responses, and Rheumatoid Arthritis," *Seminars on Arthritis and Rheumatism* 25, no. 2 (October 1995): 87–96.

were the only group to show significant improvement in both their own assessment of pain as well as that of the evaluating physicians. Furthermore, this group was able to lower their use of standard antirheumatic medicine more than the other two groups. This well-designed study provides good evidence to recommend omega-3 fatty acids for rheumatoid arthritis.[2]

New Prescription Therapies for Rheumatoid Arthritis

There are three soon-to-be-released prescription items that hold significant promise for those suffering from rheumatoid arthritis. These are the COX-II inhibitors, type II collagen, TNF antagonists, and minocycline (minocycline is discussed in chapter 9).

COX-II inhibitors
Unlike the standard NSAIDs that indiscriminately inhibit the enzyme family cyclooxygenase (COX), COX-II inhibitors selectively block only one kind of cyclooxygenase, the one associated with forming inflammation-causing prostaglandins in the body. By leaving the "good" COX-I alone, many of the side effects that are seen with the standard NSAIDs are avoided. Long-term safety data remains to be published, but these drugs look very promising.

Type II Collagen
There are fourteen types of collagen in humans. Type II is the kind found in articular (or hyaline) cartilage, the main site of attack of most forms of arthritis. It is usually derived from the articular cartilage on the ends of chicken bones and processed into a powder.

Type II is an interesting and tricky product in that injectable and oral forms have almost opposite effects. In arthritis research, animals are given laboratory-induced inflammatory arthritis by an injection of a type II collagen (mixed with other components) directly into their joints. The type II collagen is perceived as a foreign protein and rejected by the joints, resulting in a type of arthritis that is similar to rheumatoid arthritis in humans.

The oral form of type II collagen has the opposite effect. In both animals and humans *who already have* an inflammatory type of arthritis, oral type II collagen desensitizes the immune reaction and slows the body's attack on the joints. This is similar to the desensitization procedures performed by an allergist. For example, allergists give small quantities of cat dander to an individual allergic to cats. Over time, the patient develops a *tolerance* to the cat dander and does not suffer so severely the next time he or she comes in contact with cats.

Results from preliminary studies are encouraging. One report published in *Science*[3] tested the effects of type II collagen on sixty people suffering from severe rheumatoid arthritis. The participants were taken off any immunosuppressive drugs they were taking and examined. Then they were divided into two groups. Group 1 received 0.1 mg solubilized type II collagen a day for one month. That dosage was increased to 0.5 milligrams per day for the next two months. Group 2 was given a placebo.

Everyone was examined at the beginning of the ninety-day study, at the one- and two-month marks, and at the end. This was a classic double-blind study in that neither the volunteers nor the researchers knew who was receiving the collagen and who was getting the placebo until the end of the study.

The results were impressive. Those receiving collagen enjoyed significant improvement in their symptoms. The number of swollen and/or tender joints was reduced, and the degree of swelling or tenderness fell. Fourteen percent of those receiving the collagen had ''complete resolution of their disease,'' compared to 0 percent in the placebo group. The

3. D. E. Trentham et al., ''Effects of Oral Administration of Type II Collagen on Rheumatoid Arthritis.'' *Science* 2 (September 24, 1991) Vol. 261: 1727–1730.

researchers concluded that taking type II collagen "is both safe and can improve the clinical manifestations of active rheumatoid arthritis."

There are no reported significant side effects from oral type II collagen. Type II collagen in powdered form is encapsulated and taken by mouth. We believe that it may offer significant hope for the future.

TNF antagonists

Though the exact trigger for rheumatoid arthritis is not known, the inflammation that persists is due in part to a substance produced by the body called *tumor necrosis factor,* or TNF. Arthritis researchers have found that substances that counteract the action of TNF have a dramatic effect on those with rheumatoid arthritis, even in patients who do not respond well to other therapies (so-called refractory cases).

A study published in the *New England Journal of Medicine*[4] detailed a clinical trial using a genetically engineered TNF antagonist (named TNFR:Fc, trade-name Enbrel) compared to placebo on 180 subjects with refractory rheumatoid arthritis. TNFR:Fc or a placebo was injected subcutaneously twice a week for three months. The treated groups showed significant improvements in morning stiffness, pain, and tenderness in their joints compared to the placebo group. In addition, those receiving the higher doses (three different doses were used) of TNFR:Fc showed the greatest improvement, 61 percent versus 25 percent over those getting the placebo. Best of all was the tolerability of this injectable treatment—only one person dropped out of the study due to adverse reactions (tenderness at the site of injection).

TNFR:Fc is still considered to be experimental and is not yet available for general use. This drug represents a significant advance in the use of genetically derived treatments.

4. Treatment of Rheumatoid Arthritis with a Recombinant Human Tumor Necrosis Factor Receptor (p75)-Fc Fusion Protein *N Engl J Med* 337(3): 141–147 (1997).

Arava (leflunomide)

This is the most exciting of the new prescription drugs since it can help prevent joint destruction. Approved by the FDA in September 1998, Arava (generic name, leflunomide) is the first of a new class of drugs. Known as a pryimidine synthesis inhibitor, Arava is thought to act early in the disease process, blocking the build-up of cells that cause inflammation.

Arava is indicated for use in adults who have active rheumatoid arthritis. Used to reduce signs and symptoms of RA, Arava also appears to retard joint destruction as well or better than the current first-line therapy for severe RA, the antimetabolite Methotrexate. Methotrexate also works by blocking immune cell accumulation, but targets a different enzyme than Arava. Arava appears to have a better side-effect profile than does Methotrexate (which can cause kidney and liver damage). Nevertheless, about one-fourth of those receiving Arava have side effects, which include diarrhea, rash, and hair loss. Since Arava can cause birth defects, caution is needed when used in women of child-bearing age. Blood tests to monitor the liver are performed during treatment with Arava.

Conclusion

To summarize, applying our *Maximizing the Arthritis Cure* program will help you if you have rheumatoid arthritis. Research using glucosamine and chondroitin for rheumatoid arthritis is still lacking, but the positive case reports keep piling in. Anti-inflammatory oils are widely available and well tolerated. The COX-II and TNF antagonists will help with pain, and both have a low incidence of side effects. The really good news is the anti-inflammatory enzymes and the new drug, Arava. These substances offer new hope for RA sufferers everywhere.

9

Other Treatments:
What's Hype, What's Not

From the time the first caveman groaned about his aching joints, standard therapies, alternative approaches, and folk remedies for osteoarthritis have abounded. Some relieve pain, some work on inflammation, and some appear to help the body heal itself. Some work well, but only for certain people. Others are probably helpful, but we haven't yet figured out exactly how they work, and their value hasn't been demonstrated in enough scientific studies to make them generally acceptable. Then there are those that have no therapeutic value whatsoever. Since the symptoms of osteoarthritis naturally wax and wane, the disease is a prime candidate for treatments that appear to work, but don't pan out when carefully studied. But how do you know what's real and what's not? Let this chapter serve as your guide. For each of the "remedies" discussed, we provide a definition of what it is, why it's used, whether it works, if it has any known side effects, and how it's normally administered or taken. But a word of caution before we begin.

A Warning

Some of the new products coming onto the market may help you fight arthritis. However, health is an area that seems to attract charlatans. So we urge you to maintain a level of healthy suspicion toward any treatment you are considering. The warning signs that things may not be on the up and up are:

- Information on a given product is available only from a manufacturer, distributor, or promoter of a product and not from a university or independent academic resource or peer-reviewed journal. Some companies overstate or inaccurately report "medical" information on a product. In the worst case, they literally make up information about a product.
- The product claims to work on an inordinate number of conditions, such as all (100) forms of arthritis. Very few treatments in medicine work on more than a few, generally related, conditions.
- The claims of efficacy are based on "proof" from testimonials of individual patients or even healthcare providers.
- Only one scientific study is quoted for evidence, with no confirmatory studies performed by an independent group. The hallmark of the scientific theory is to have an independent organization duplicate the study and come up with the same or similar findings.
- A study is cited that does not have a control group. Without a control, you cannot be sure the results were not merely the placebo effect in action. Some people do better just by being in a study even if they receive no treatment.
- The product is based on a "special" or "secret" formula. If something truly works, companies are the first ones to toot their own horn and tell everyone what's in the product, so they can get credit for their success.
- The product does not have a complete listing of ingredients. For example, beware of the word *complex* if specific

amounts are not listed. A manufacturer stating that a product contains a certain amount of chondroitin/glucosamine "complex" may be selling you 95 percent glucosamine (the cheaper of the two ingredients) and only 5 percent chondroitin.

• The product supposedly contains the same ingredients as supplements manufactured by other companies, though the product in question is substantially lower priced than nearly all other brands. The manufacturers may be able to do this because the bulk of the nutrient/product they are using is so impure that ingesting it results in little therapeutic effect. (Of course, the opposite is not true: Just because a product is overpriced does not mean that it is purer or better. Some manufacturers overprice simply because some people will overpay.)

Boswellia (Boswellin)

WHAT IS IT?
Boswellia Serrata is a tree native to India. From this tree comes a gum resin called *salai guggul*.

WHY IS IT USED?
In animal studies, *salai guggul* has been shown to inhibit inflammation and prevent the loss of glycosaminoglycans, which are important proteins found in cartilage.[1]

DOES IT WORK?
Unfortunately, there is little substantive human research and other supporting information on *boswellia*, making it impossible to make definitive statements about its therapeutic value.

1. G. B. Singh, and C. K. Atal, "Pharmacology of an Extract of Salai Guggul Ex-Boswellia Serrata, a New Non-Steroidal Anti-Inflammatory Agent," *Agents Action* 18 (1986): 407–12; C. K. Reddy, et al., "Studies on the Metabolism of Glycosaminoglycans Under the Influence of New Herbal Anti-Inflammatory Agent," *Biochemical Pharmacology* 20 (1989): 3527–34.

WHAT ARE ITS SIDE EFFECTS?
No side effects from boswellic acids have been reported.

HOW IS IT TAKEN?
Boswellia is usually ground into a powder and taken orally. Like many herbs that are not standardized in their potency, the safe and effective dosage is not known.

Capsaicin

WHAT IS IT?
Pronounced "cap-SAY-shun," it's the "hot stuff" in chili peppers. Capsaicin lotion or cream has been used to help relieve arthritis and other pains. Formerly a prescription item, it is now available over the counter in different strengths.

WHY IS IT USED?
To treat the pain of osteo- and other forms of arthritis. Additionally, it's used for the treatment of pain from shingles. Capsaicin is just a pain reliever and does not appear to have any disease-modifying effects. People often use capsaicin for mild to moderate joint pain, especially of the fingers, hands, wrists, and knees, essentially anywhere the joints are close to the surface and easily accessible. Some people use capsaicin because they have only one or two painful small joints and don't feel the need to take pills for pain control. Capsaicin is also used as an adjunct to other treatments for arthritis.

DOES IT WORK?
There's much we don't yet know about capsaicin and pain. Capsaicin seems to act on a chemical in your nervous system responsible for sending pain messages from the nerve endings in your joints and surrounding tissues to the brain. This chemical, called substance P (the *P* stands for *pain*), is depleted from the nerve endings, essentially blocking transmission of the pain signal. Capsaicin may also have the effect of reducing inflammation in rheumatoid arthritis.

WHAT ARE ITS SIDE EFFECTS?
The only significant side effect reported is stinging or burning at the application site. This is usually temporary. Failure to wash your hands after application can lead to burning in your eyes or other sensitive areas, if you inadvertently touch them.

HOW IS IT TAKEN?
Capsaicin is applied topically, directly over the affected joints. It must be used three to four times per day and it seems to take at least a few days and as much as a month before its effect really kicks in. This delay is presumably due to the time it takes to deplete substance P from the nerve endings. Capsaicin is never ingested by mouth, and eating chili peppers does not give the same effect as topically applying it.

Cat's Claw

WHAT IS IT?
Also known as *uña de gato,* cat's claw is an Amazonian herb that belongs to a class of compounds known as *quinovic acid glycosides* that are thought to have some anti-inflammatory properties.

WHY IS IT USED?
To treat inflammation and pain in several different types of arthritis and other conditions causing inflammation.

DOES IT WORK?
There is no good information to suggest that cat's claw is effective for treating arthritis pain or inflammation.

WHAT ARE ITS SIDE EFFECTS?
The side effect profile is not well established.

HOW IS IT TAKEN?
It is usually made into a powdered form and mixed into a capsule containing other herbs, or it can be brewed as a tea.

Devil's Claw

WHAT IS IT?
Devil's claw—its Latin name is *Harpagophytum procumbens*—is a plant native to South Africa. The root of the plant is used for its medicinal benefit.

WHY IS IT USED?
It's used to reduce pain and inflammation.

DOES IT WORK?
Devil's claw has been put to the test in some small scientific studies, but there is not enough proof to establish that it effectively alleviates the symptoms of osteoarthritis.

WHAT ARE ITS SIDE EFFECTS?
Although devil's claw appears to have no significant side effects with short-term use, we don't know what will happen if it's taken for long periods of time.

HOW IS IT TAKEN?
Devil's claw is usually taken in capsule, liquid, or dry-solid form, or as a powder added to tea. The popular dosage is 100 mg per day of 5 percent standardized extract.

DMSO (Dimethyl Sulfoxide)

WHAT IS IT?
Used as an industrial solvent since the 1940s, DMSO is derived from lignin (found in wood). DMSO wasn't used therapeutically until the 1960s. It is approved for use as an anti-inflammatory in horses.

WHY IS IT USED?
DMSO is used to reduce the inflammation of swollen joints and as a penetrant to increase the absorption of medications through the skin.

WHAT ARE ITS SIDE EFFECTS?
Although DMSO is colorless and odorless, once applied to the skin it may leave your breath smelling of garlic or onions. And it has been shown to cause damage to the lens of the eye in animal studies. In humans it can be potentially toxic to the liver, as well. The most common side effects are skin rashes, headache, nausea, and diarrhea.

HOW IS IT TAKEN?
DMSO is applied externally to the skin. *We do not recommend its use,* since there are safer alternatives.

Feverfew

WHAT IS IT?
Feverfew, the Latin name for which is *Tanacetum parthenium,* is a plant native to Germany, Holland, the UK, and Israel. The leaves of the plant are harvested and extracted. The extract is then standardized for potency in terms of how much parthenolide (an active component) it contains.

WHY IS IT USED?
It's used to reduce pain and inflammation.

DOES IT WORK?
There is not enough definitive proof to establish that it effectively alleviates the symptoms of osteoarthritis, but it can help with the pain from inflammatory conditions. People often report that it takes up to a month to notice the effects from taking feverfew.

WHAT ARE ITS SIDE EFFECTS?
Although feverfew appears to have no significant side effects with short-term use, we don't know what will happen if it's taken for long periods of time.

How Is It Taken?
Feverfew is taken in capsule, the dosage is 500 mg/day of extract standardized to contain parthenolide 0.1–0.5 percent, one of feverfew's active components.

Ginger

What Is It?
A popular seasoning, ginger root has been used for almost two thousand years to treat different ailments, including fever, diarrhea, and vomiting. Recent scientific studies suggest that it may help prevent heart disease by "thinning" the blood.

Why Is It Used?
Today, ginger is used as a remedy for heartburn, indigestion, vomiting, and motion sickness. Some have suggested that it might also be helpful for arthritis.

Does It Work?
It appears to help many people with motion sickness and indigestion. There is as yet no convincing evidence, however, that the herb helps relieve or reverse osteoarthritis. Ginger has been shown to have some anti-inflammatory effects similar to NSAIDs (by inhibiting the enzyme cyclooxygenase).

What Are Its Side Effects?
Ginger is generally well tolerated, although ingesting large amounts may cause the heart to beat irregularly and may slightly suppress the central nervous system. In the 1930s, an alcoholic beverage made from Jamaican ginger caused a neurological disorder called the Jake Walk in some people. Taking excess ginger may interfere to a small extent with the absorption of certain nutrients. Pregnant and nursing women should consult their physicians before taking large amounts of the herb—and before making any decisions that will affect their health.

HOW IS IT TAKEN?
Fresh or in capsules containing 500 mg per day. Powdered or dry ginger, 1.5 grams per day. It is also available as candied ginger, ginger beer, or ginger tea.

Nettles

WHAT ARE THEY?
Nettles (or stinging nettles), the Latin name for which is *Urtica dioica*, are plants native to Europe and Israel. The leaves of young plants are harvested and extracted. The extract is then standardized for the potency of the plant silica it contains.

WHY ARE THEY USED?
They're used to reduce pain and inflammation. Nettles are also used as a vitamin and mineral supplement since they contain magnesium, silica, potassium, sulfur, and vitamins A, C, B_2, and B_5 (in addition to several phytochemicals).

DO THEY WORK?
Nettles have a long history of use in the treatment of gout and other rheumatic conditions but have not been studied specifically for osteoarthritis.

WHAT ARE THEIR SIDE EFFECTS?
Although nettles appear to have no significant side effects with short-term use, we don't know what happens if they are taken for long periods.

HOW ARE THEY TAKEN?
Nettles are taken in capsule form. The dosage is 750 mg per day of extract standardized to contain 1–2 percent plant silica.

Niacinamide

WHAT IS IT?
Niacinamide is a form of Vitamin B_3, the water-soluble vitamin that helps the body produce energy and keeps body cells functioning properly.

WHY IS IT USED?
Niacinamide is used to improve joint function.

DOES IT WORK?
It has been shown to improve joint mobility when used in high doses.[2] However, the studies supporting niacinamide date back to the mid- to late 1950s, and we are unaware of significant follow-up studies that prove or disprove these findings. It appears that in order for niacinamide to be effective on an ongoing basis, it must be taken frequently and for the long term.[3] It is generally not used to treat arthritis by today's physicians.

WHAT ARE ITS SIDE EFFECTS?
High doses of niacinamide may damage the liver.

HOW IS IT TAKEN?
Niacinamide is taken orally.

2. W. Kaufman, "The Use of Vitamin Therapy to Reduce Certain Concomitants of Aging," *Journal of the American Geriatric Society* 3 (1955): 927; A. Hoffer, "Treatment of Osteoarthritis by Nicotinic Acid and Nicotinamide," *Canadian Medical Association Journal*, Canadian Medical Society 8fl (1959): 235–39.
3. L. Bucci, *Nutrition Applied to Injury Rehabilitation and Sports Medicine* (Boca Raton, FL: CRC Press, 1994), p. 88.

Shark Cartilage

WHAT IS IT?
Shark cartilage is made up of extracts derived from the carti-laginous skeletons of one or more of the dozens of species of sharks.

WHY IS IT USED?
It is often used as a replacement to chondroitin sulfate. Also, it is being studied as an anticancer agent, though preliminary data for this particular use do not seem to be very positive.

DOES IT WORK?
Although preliminary anecdotal and clinical experience sug-gests that shark cartilage may be helpful in certain cases, it is still too early to state definitively that it has significant thera-peutic value in treating osteoarthritis. If it does, it is probably because it contains small amounts of glucosamine and chon-droitin. The amount of glucosamine and chondroitin in shark cartilage is very low, however, and the chondroitin may be of a different variety from the one proved to have effect in treat-ing arthritis. Shark cartilage, because of its low yield of glu-cosamine and chondroitin, is a very expensive and imprecise way to obtain these nutrients. We are confident that it is much better to take these supplements in regular pill forms, not as shark cartilage.

WHAT ARE ITS SIDE EFFECTS?
No side effects have been reported from this widely used prod-uct. We do not yet have enough information to state whether there are any long-term adverse effects, however. Products on the market are taken from many sources and are not carefully controlled by many of their manufacturers. Some of the sharks used may be contaminated with heavy metals, such as mer-cury, and organic toxins, such as PCBs. Sharks, being at the top of the ocean's food chain, are more prone to accumulating toxins through their diet.

How Is It Taken?
In pill or powder form.

Superoxide Dismutase (SOD)

What Is It?
SOD is an enzyme frequently extracted from bovine liver for its use in supplement form. It's found in most human and mammal cells.

Why Is It Used?
SOD is used to control inflammation and free radicals.

Does It Work?
In test tube studies, SOD has scavenged free radical substances, such as superoxide and hydroxyl radicals, that harm tissue and may contribute to the cartilage damage seen in osteoarthritis. Some studies on humans using injectable SOD have shown that it can help reduce inflammation, while others have been inconclusive.

What Are Its Side Effects?
Years of clinical use have not revealed any significant side effects. Bear in mind, though, that whenever you inject something into a joint there is a minor risk of infection.

How Is It Taken?
SOD is administered by injection, usually directly into the affected joint. Oral SOD doesn't appear to be of any benefit since it is broken down by the body's gastrointestinal system before it can get into the joints.

Turmeric

What Is It?
Turmeric, the Latin name for which is *Curcuma longa,* is a plant native to India that is used as a spice in Indian and other

ethnic cuisines. It often provides the yellow color to curry dishes. The rhizome (part of the root system) is harvested, and the extract is then standardized for the potency of curcumin (its active component) it contains.

WHY IS IT USED?
Turmeric, or more specifically its active ingredient curcumin, has anti-inflammatory properties, some of which are similar to those of NSAIDs. It also has some antioxidant properties. It is used to treat the pain and inflammation of osteo- and other forms of arthritis. It is also used as an adjunct to the four ACES.

DOES IT WORK?
Turmeric has a long history of use in the treatment of inflammatory conditions, but it has not been studied specifically for use in osteoarthritis.

WHAT ARE ITS SIDE EFFECTS?
Turmeric appears to have no significant side effects with short-term use, but we don't know what happens if it's taken for long periods of time. Avoid doses above 300 mg per day if you have liver or gallbladder problems, such as gallstones.

HOW IS IT TAKEN?
When used "medically," turmeric is taken with meals, in 100-mg capsules. Take a product that is standardized to 95 percent curcumin.

Tetracycline/Doxycycline/Minocycline

WHAT ARE THEY?
These are all prescription antibiotics in the tetracycline family. Tetracycline is the original in this group, with doxycycline and minocycline being analogs. Minocycline has received a lot of attention lately following a promising study conducted by the University of Nebraska with rheumatoid arthritis patients.

WHY ARE THEY USED?

Tetracycline and its analogs are approved for use in animals and are currently being studied for human use in treating rheumatoid arthritis. Rheumatologists interviewed by the AP believe that minocycline may soon be widely prescribed. These drugs are believed to work in at least one of three ways:

- As anti-inflammatory agents, using a different mechanism from NSAIDs.
- As antimicrobial agents. One theory on the development of rheumatoid arthritis is that victims have or had a bacterial or parasitic infection that may be, at least in part, treatable with certain antibiotics.
- To inhibit degrading enzymes, specifically of the metalloproteinases (enzymes produced by chondrocytes that break down cartilage).

WHAT ARE THEIR SIDE EFFECTS?

All of the usual side effects of antibiotics, such as stomach upset, diarrhea, yeast infections, drug allergies, medication interactions, and the potential for creating drug-resistant strains of bacteria, are possible reactions. Enhanced sunburn response is a classic side effect of tetracycline analogs.

HOW ARE THEY ADMINISTERED?

As pills, in low doses. These drugs do not yet have FDA approval for treating human arthritis, but they soon may become a standard treatment. A physician's prescription is required.

External Treatments

Let's take a look now at several of the popular treatments for osteoarthritis that are not in the form of ingestables but are administered outside the body. Mainstream physicians and health professionals offer several of these therapies, while others are available only through alternative healers.

A note of caution: Some of these therapies can be dangerous even when offered by mainstream physicians. So be sure to ask the questions listed in this chapter before agreeing to any kind of treatment. And make sure that any treatment you undergo is monitored by your regular physician.

Acupressure

WHAT IS IT?
Acupressure is a traditional method of Chinese healing. Using their hands (and sometimes feet), acupressurists apply firm pressure to certain points on the body in order to release tension and increase blood circulation.

WHY IS IT USED?
Acupressure is used to relieve pain.

DOES IT WORK?
It has helped relieve the joint pain of many osteoarthritis sufferers; however most report that the pain relief is very short-lived. Applying pressure to special points on the body relaxes the muscles and may cause pain nerve fibers to be compressed, which in turn helps to relieve pain.

WHAT ARE ITS SIDE EFFECTS?
There are no known side effects to acupressure when it is properly applied.

HOW IS IT ADMINISTERED?
The acupressurist applies a steady, firm pressure to certain "acupoints" on the body. Hundreds of these special points are found all over our bodies, most of them just below major muscle groups, joints, or in the hollows of bones.

Acupuncture

WHAT IS IT?
A part of traditional Chinese medicine, acupuncture uses very tiny needles inserted at specific points in the body to stimulate and balance the flow of vital energy, *qi* (pronounced "chee") in the body, release tension, and increase circulation.

WHY IS IT USED?
It's used to relieve the pain associated with osteoarthritis and to restore vital energy according to Asian medicine practitioners. Eastern medical philosophy holds that disruption of these energy patterns is the cause of illness.

DOES IT WORK?
Acupuncture relieves osteoarthritis symptoms for many people. There are some good studies showing the benefits of acupuncture for combating arthritis pain. For example, in a study conducted at the University of Maryland School of Medicine, patients with osteoarthritis of the knee enjoyed temporary relief from pain, and increased mobility in the joint(s), after receiving acupuncture twice a week for eight weeks. We don't know exactly why it works (from a Western science standpoint), and it doesn't necessarily work for everyone. One theory holds that it stimulates the body to produce more endorphins, the "feel good" hormones that are known to block pain. Another is that healing actually improves when the balance of *qi* is restored to the affected joint(s).

WHAT ARE ITS SIDE EFFECTS?
There are no known significant side effects to acupuncture when it is administered properly by a certified professional acupuncturist. Rarely, a needle may lead to bleeding or infection. There have been some cases of misplacement of a needle into a nerve, leading to local pain or sensory changes.

How Is It Administered?
Needles are carefully inserted through the skin in certain areas
of the body, some at the site of the pain, others a distance
away. The needles may be twirled as they are put in place, or
attached to wires that allow a very low-voltage current to be
delivered through the needles in order to amplify the therapeutic benefit.

The American Academy of Medical Acupuncture (800-521-
2262) can help refer you to a physician who has had at least
two hundred hours of training in acupuncture.

Biomagnetic Therapy

What Is It?
There are two types of biomagnetic therapy. One type is generated from electromagnets and is known as Pulsed Electromagnetic Field Therapy (PEMF); the other is generated from
permanent therapeutic magnets. PEMF and permanent magnets are different in some important ways. Although both have
been shown to have a salutary effect on pain, far more research
has been conducted on PEMF, and it is now widely used in
hospitals.

Fixed field, permanent therapeutic magnets are similar to
standard refrigerator magnets except that they are considerably
stronger. They are affixed to each painful part of the body
with Velcro straps, or other types of wraps, and are worn usually for a few hours or more. Alternatively, they may also
work when affixed over acupressure points in the body. Some
people sleep on mattresses, drive on car seats, or wear shoe
insoles containing permanent magnets. The Miami Dolphins
have a magnetized mat covering the bench on which players
rest while they are not in the game.

Why Is It Used?
PEMF is widely used in hospitals to lessen pain, facilitate the
knitting of bones, and speed the healing of wounds.

Permanent magnets are used by many people to treat joint

pain and inflammation, and a number of newspaper articles have appeared lately indicating that some professional golfers and football players use permanent magnets to relieve back and neck pain. In Japan, an estimated 75 percent of all households use permanent magnets to relieve various types of pain.

Does It Work?

PEMF has been shown to be effective in alleviating pain, and a number of placebo-controlled studies have been performed. In context with arthritis, there have been two clinical trials using a double-blind, randomized protocol and placebo control. In the first, twenty-seven patients with osteoarthritis, primarily of the knee, were treated with PEMF. The results showed an average improvement in decreased pain and improved function of 23–61 percent for those receiving the actual treatment, versus 2–18 percent improvement for those in the placebo group.[4] In the more recent study, eighty-six patients with osteoarthritis of the knee and eighty-one with osteoarthritis of the cervical spine received eighteen half-hour PEMF or placebo treatments. Patients were evaluated for the reduction in pain, pain on passive motion, and joint tenderness. Evaluations were made by the patient and an examining physician. The results showed impressive improvement from the baseline, leading the researchers to conclude that PEMF has therapeutic benefit in painful osteoarthritis of the knee and cervical spine.[5]

Permanent magnets are also known to relieve many different types of pain as shown by numerous studies, some of

4. D. H. Trock, A. J. Bollet, R. H. Dyer, L. P. Fielding, W. K. Miner, and R. Markoli, "A Double-Blind Trial of the Clinical Effects of Pulsed Electromagnetic fields in Osteoarthritis," *J Rheumatol* 20 (1994): 456–60.

5. D. H. Trock, A. J. Bollet, R. H. Dyer, L. P. Fielding, W. K. Miner, and R. Markoli, "The Effect of Pulsed Electromagnetic Fields in the Treatment of Osteoarthritis of the Knee and Cervical Spine, Report of Randomized, Double-Blind, Placebo Controlled Trials," *J Rheumatol* 21, no. 10 (October 1994): 1903–11.

which are referenced below.[6] There have been no studies, however, that have studied the effects of permanent magnets on the pain caused by arthritis. Nevertheless, we feel comfortable in suggesting you try them for yourself.

WHAT ARE ITS SIDE EFFECTS?
There are no known side effects from fixed magnets.

Electromagnetic fields, such as those generated by the electricity flowing through power lines, have been accused of causing many health problems, including cancer and childhood leukemia. Such studies led to near-panic among some owners of homes located near high-tension power lines. A recent, very thorough, study has found no validity to these rumors. The magnetic fields generated by power lines, microwaves, and electrical appliances do not cause leukemia. Moreover, since these magnetic fields are considerably weaker than the magnetic fields generated by Earth itself, it appears that they would be too weak to do this type of harm.

On the other hand, the electromagnetic fields generated for certain therapeutic purposes are far more powerful than permanent magnets. Although no serious negative side effects have been observed, such treatments should be under medical supervision and handled with care.

HOW IS IT ADMINISTERED?
PEMF therapy is usually administered in a hospital or clinic where patients insert their sore joints into an electromagnetic device, usually for half-hour sessions, several times a week.

6. Vallbona, Hazlewood, Jurida, "Response of Pain to Static Magnetic fields in Postpolio Patients: A Double Blind Piolet Study," *Arch Phys Med Rehabil*, Vol. 78 (November 1997): 1200–1203; Kyoichi Nakagawa, "Magnetic Field Deficiency Syndrome and Magnetic Treatment," *Japan Medical Journal* (December 4, 1976): 2745; C. Takeshige, and M. Sato, "Comparison of Pain Relief Mechanism Between Needling to the Muscle, Static Magnetic Field, External *Qigong* and Needling to the Acupuncture Point," *Acupuncture and Electro-Therapeutics Research* (1996) 21(no. 2): 119–131; K. S. Kim and Y. J. Lee. "The Effect of Magnetic Application for Primary Dysmenorrhea," *Kanhohak Tamgu* 3, no. 1 (1994): 148–173.

The treatment typically lasts a number of weeks. One study indicates that longer treatments may be more effective. Some portable devices are available. One of the research studies used a portable device that was worn six to ten hours per day, including while asleep.

Permanent magnets are worn on the affected joint continuously, held in place with either elastic or Velcro devices. The magnets come in different shapes and sizes to fit comfortably on the painful areas.

Cold Therapy

WHAT IS IT?
A variety of treatments that apply cold to the body, including such treatments as cold baths, ice, cold gel-packs (that mold around a joint), and even simple household items like a bag of frozen peas or beans.

WHY IS IT USED?
Cold therapy has both anti-inflammatory and analgesic (pain-relieving) properties. Ice, with compression, is perhaps the most powerful means of relieving swelling in and around a joint.

DOES IT WORK?
Yes, very well, but the relief is usually only short-lived.

WHAT ARE ITS SIDE EFFECTS?
Leaving a cold object on the skin too long can actually cause the skin to freeze. On certain parts of the body, like the inside of the elbow and outside of the knee, prolonged exposure to cold could damage one of the superficially located nerves in the area (the ulnar nerve and common peroneal nerve, respectively).

How Is It Administered?
A cold object is placed over the affected area for ten to fifteen minutes. A thin cloth between the skin and the cold is recommended to avoid freezing the skin.

Electrical Stimulation

What Is It?
Electrical stimulation is, as it sounds, the application of small doses of electricity to specific parts of the body. It's also known as Transcutaneous Electrical Nerve Stimulation, or TENS for short.

Why Is It Used?
TENS is used to alleviate the pain associated with osteoarthritis. It is a well-established modality for treatment of various types of chronic pain.

Does It Work?
Some have experienced pain relief from the treatment; others have not. When it works, it quells pain for anywhere from a few hours to a few days. However, TENS usually becomes less and less effective over time, and there is no evidence that TENS has any curative effect.

What Are Its Side Effects?
There are no known side effects from this therapy when properly applied.

How Is It Administered?
Special electrodes are coated with a gel and attached to the skin on or near the affected area. The electrodes are attached by wires to the TENS unit, which sends low-level electricity into the skin (using a nine-volt battery) through the wires and electrodes. Patients may feel a tingling sensation, or feel nothing at all.

Heat Therapy

WHAT IS IT?
This therapy includes a variety of treatments that apply heat to the body. These include hot baths, hot compresses, whirlpools, showers, heat lamps, heating pads, heating mitts, and paraffin wax treatments.

WHY IS IT USED?
Heat is used to relax muscles and reduce joint pain.

DOES IT WORK?
Yes. Heat has helped countless numbers of people by temporarily reducing or relieving pain while improving a joint's range of motion. Heat has no permanent curative effect.

WHAT ARE ITS SIDE EFFECTS?
Properly applied, heat treatments have no side effects. They are not, however, indicated for acute injuries or inflammation, which it may worsen. Also, you may encounter difficulty from full-body heat treatment (for example, saunas) if you have certain preexisting conditions that limit or prohibit the application of heat. For example, if you have heart disease or are on certain medications, you should strictly limit your time in warm whirlpools and hot baths—or refrain from them altogether—to avoid fatigue and the dangers that may occur in these locales. Check with your physician before undergoing such heat treatments.

HOW IS IT USED?
A heating pad, lamp, or other object is placed on or above the affected area or part, or all of the body is immersed in heated water or in a steam sauna. (Moist heat tends to penetrate deeper.)

Topical Analgesic Creams

WHAT IS IT?
These are creams you buy over the counter that often contain aspirin and other products that deliver heat to the skin and surrounding tissues. The aspirin (or other anti-inflammatory) gets absorbed locally and can relieve pain.

WHY IS IT USED?
To relieve muscle and joint pain.

DOES IT WORK?
Yes, these usually provide relief for mild osteoarthritis pain, especially in joints that are close to the surface of the skin, such as fingers, knuckles, elbows and knees. Usually, the relief is short-lived.

WHAT ARE THE SIDE EFFECTS?
None. Just be sure to wash your hands after use to avoid getting any in your eyes.

HOW IS IT TAKEN?
Usually a cream consists of methylsalicylate 15–30 percent with menthol 10 percent and camphor 4 percent along with other ingredients. The cream is typically applied to the affected joint one to three times per day.

A "Special" Treatment

A great deal has been written about the mind-body connection in the past two decades. Some of its seems like science fiction—until you read the serious, scientific studies that support it. A new branch of medicine, called *psychoneuroimmunology,* has recently arisen, probing and chronicling the mind-body relationship. This new field is offering us an entirely new way to look at and use the mind as medicine.

In an interesting study that confirmed the influence of the mind over the immune system,[7] researchers at the University of California at Los Angeles asked actors to act "happy" and "sad" scenes. To see how pretending to be happy or sad was influencing the actors' immune systems, the researchers took saliva samples to measure the T-cell proliferation rate, an indication of immune system strength. The results? When the actors acted happy, their T-cell proliferation rate rose, indicating that their immune systems were stronger. When they acted sad, the rate dropped, reflecting weakness in the immune system. All it took was *acting* happy or sad to influence the immune system.

This has tremendous implications for chronic pain patients, including arthritis sufferers, many of whom understandably become sad, frustrated, angry, or depressed. These unhappy emotions may be weakening their immune systems, putting them at higher risk of developing various diseases, suffering more, and becoming progressively more unhappy. Clearly, breaking the cycle of unhappiness is important. Instead of sadness, pain patients need something positive to look forward to, something that will strengthen their immune systems and possibly help to ease their pain.

That something does not have to be what we normally think of as a medicine. In a fascinating test of the mind-body connection,[8] thirty-two patients were gathered by scientists at the University of Tennessee Center for Health Sciences. These patients, suffering from intractable back pain, had not been helped by standard therapies. The researchers began by measuring the levels of endorphins in the patients' spinal fluid. (Endorphins are natural hormones that, among other things, regulate pain in the body. They are, in a sense, our "internal

7. As reported by A. Fox and B. Fox, *Beyond Positive Thinking* (Carson, CA: Hay House, 1991), p. 64.

8. J. J. Lippman, et al., "CSF Endorphin Levels in Chronic Pain Patients Before and After Placebo Pain relief," in *Advances in Endogenous and Exogenous Opioids: Proceedings of the International Narcotic Research Conference*, ed. H. Takagi and E. J. Simon (Tokyo: Kodansha, 1981), pp. 315–17.

morphine,'' an integral part of our built-in pain control system.)

Having measured the endorphins, the scientists then gave the patients placebos with no medicinal value. Fourteen of the thirty-two patients (44 percent) soon reported feeling better.

That's interesting, but this is the amazing part: When the scientists remeasured the endorphin levels in those fourteen, they found that the levels had risen. It was the endorphins that were blocking the patients' pain, but what caused the endorphin levels to rise? Since a placebo has no physiological effect, clearly it was the patients' belief—their simple conviction that they would soon be healed—that bumped up their endorphin levels. They believed they would feel better, their positive thoughts were ''converted'' into endorphins, and their pain was quelled.

These and other studies have confirmed that positive thinking, believing you are going to get well, can help strengthen the immune system, reduce pain, and sometimes even help to prolong life. One report in *The Journal of the American Medical Association*[9] found that the death rate among Jewish men fell significantly before Passover. When the holiday was over, the death rate jumped to above normal, as if to compensate for those who perhaps ''should'' have died during Passover, then settled back to normal. Somehow, some of these men ''slated'' for death managed to postpone the fatal event until the holiday had passed. A similar phenomenon was observed among elderly Chinese women shortly before the Harvest Moon Festival, a holiday with special symbolic significance for older Chinese women.

We can't say exactly how these men and women managed possibly to postpone their deaths, but we do know that they were looking forward to these holidays with positive anticipation. The same kind of positive thinking has proved to increase endorphin levels and strengthen the immune system.

Receiving emotional support can also favorably alter a per-

9. D. P. Phillips and D. G. Smith, ''Postponement of Death Until Symbolically Meaningful Occasions,'' *JAMA* 363, no. 14 (April 11, 1990): 1947–51.

son's biochemistry. In an astonishing study conducted at Stanford University, eighty-six women with breast cancer that had spread beyond their breasts were randomly assigned to either a control or support group. The control group was given standard medical care, while the support group received standard care plus weekly support group sessions. One year later, the women in the support group were less anxious and depressed than those in the control group and felt only half as much pain. More important, the women in the support group lived longer—an average of eighteen months more than the control group. The only difference in the treatment of the two groups was that the support group had companionship, compassion, education, and mutual support. These unmeasurable, ephemeral attributes had measurable, lasting value.

Clearly, what we think can influence our health and our response to treatment. We are not suggesting that you pick any old therapy and "make" it work by believing in it, or that you throw away your medicine and simply "think health." We do suggest, however, that your attitude toward your pain, your therapy, and your odds of recovery are all an integral part of your health and healing. Believing that your therapy will work is an important part of the medicine's effectiveness. Of course, you can't force yourself to believe in something. But you can increase your positive attitude and belief by working with doctors you trust, whose knowledge you respect, and who inspire confidence. You can study the various possible therapies, looking for the one that makes sense to you. You can keep reminding yourself that you are doing everything possible to conquer your pain. You can join a support group for additional emotional aid, education, and other assistance. If you do that, you'll speed the healing process.

There's another thing you can do—laugh. Laugh out loud a couple of times every day. If nothing funny happens, just start laughing anyhow. That may seem pretty funny in itself. Even if it feels forced at first, laughter, even your own, is infectious. So give it a try. Some people say it's truly "good medicine." And it can't hurt. If regular laughing can shift the body's biochemistry in favor of health, well, that's something to smile about!

Osteoarthritis is a disease that can be largely or completely treated in a very large number of patients. The situation is improving daily. We feel confident that, for the large majority of sufferers, their problem can already be alleviated. Someday, osteoarthritis may actually be a rarity.

For those whose suffering cannot be alleviated by either the arthritis cure or the maximizing plan, and those people whose joints are so damaged that little cartilage remains, we provide a chapter on surgery. We believe you should have as much information as possible before making any health decisions, and this next chapter gives you the most recent research available on this option of last resort.

10

Curing the "Incurable": New Injectable and Surgical Techniques

"Hey, Nurse," whispered the nervous-looking twenty-eight-year-old man who was about to be wheeled into the operating room for knee surgery. "I wrote 'yes' on my right knee and 'no' on my left, just in case they have any doubt when they start cutting. Think it'll help?" Actually, some hospitals do exactly that—in one case a nurse wrote "NO WAY" on the wrong leg of a patient headed for orthoscopic knee surgery.

The fact is, surgery frightens most of us—and by and large, for good reason. After all, even the mildest surgery involves cutting into us, and it is never entirely risk-free. But, here again, we can give you some good news.

First, quite often surgery can be avoided by maximizing the arthritis cure. Of course, that is not often the first recommendation a surgeon makes. After all, surgeons are trained in surgery, they are paid to do surgery, and they *believe* in surgery, so they are likely to recommend surgery. That is not unethical. After all, you wouldn't want to be treated by surgeons who didn't believe in the value, safety, and efficacy of their art! But that doesn't mean that surgery is necessarily the best solution for you.

In fact, dozens of patients have been able to avoid surgery by following our treatment program, even ones who were told there was no choice but to operate.

Second, even if maximizing the arthritis cure is insufficient in resolving your problem, there are now far less invasive options than full surgery. Used in conjunction with glucosamine/chondroitin and the rest of our program, these options can be highly effective and often restore the function of your damaged joints. In this context, we encourage you to explore these new treatments with your doctor and then to see what treatments are available to restore your arthritic joint and thereby reduce the chances of a joint replacement later on, since restoration is often better in the long run. In any case, starting glucosamine and chondroitin therapy prior to surgery, and continuing it afterward, dramatically increases the chance of cartilage healing.

Finally, even if you decide that you do need surgery, there are now techniques that are both highly effective and very low in risk. Nevertheless, don't make that decision quickly. You need to be mentally prepared for the surgery itself and for the recovery period that may last for months. Explore all the other options before you even think of having surgery. Surgery doesn't always work, but it always carries some risk. Before agreeing to have surgery, ask yourself:

- How will this surgery make me feel better?
- What happens if the surgery fails? Will I be left disabled, or worse off than before?
- How will the surgery affect any other serious medical problems that I have?
- Will I damage another area of my body by favoring the area operated on?
- Am I too heavy (or light) for surgery? Does my weight put me at a special risk?
- Do I have an adequate support system (someone to shop, cook and clean, and offer emotional support) while I am temporarily out of commission?
- Can I accept a slow, gradual healing process? Will being

unable to take care of myself and get around upset me
greatly?
- Can I follow through with my doctor's and therapist's treatment plans? Can I wholeheartedly commit myself to the recovery process, even if it's painful, difficult, and requires a
lot of effort?
- Can I afford the time, money, and emotional investment that
this surgery requires?
- Above all, have I given the arthritis cure a fair trial? (Most
surgery can be avoided if you do.)

When they ask themselves these questions, a surprising
number of people realize that the surgeries their doctors are
recommending are simply not worth it. The benefits do not
outweigh the physical, emotional, and financial costs. The recovery process is too arduous, and the risks are too great.

On the other hand, an operation is advisable for sufferers
who have tried maximizing the arthritis cure with insufficient
success and whose pain and dysfunction are so severe that they
are chair-bound and hardly able to move. Such continuing disability is likely to lead to depression, weight gain, diabetes,
high blood pressure, excess cholesterol, and even heart disease. Moreover, some patients' health may deteriorate so much
that they later become poor candidates for an operation.

The Potential Benefits of Surgery and How to Decide If It's Right for You

The right surgery, performed by the right doctor, at the right
time, on the right joint, can work miracles—even though it
cannot replace that with which you were born. However, lining
up these four "rights" can be tricky. These are the steps you
should take to help you decide if this is the best option.

1. First, make sure that nothing else works. If this is so, you
are at least a candidate for surgery. If you have not taken

this step, we urge you to do so before even considering surgery.

2. Next, conclude, after carefully evaluating your state, that you absolutely need pain relief. The pain from your arthritis is so bad that it truly interferes with the quality of your life. People who are in constant pain may simply feel that life isn't worthwhile. It's hard to be happy when you hurt. Anger, depression, loss of sleep, and just giving up are typical side effects of chronic pain. If that circumstance applies to you, surgery is worth a try. The pain relief can be dramatic after a successful operation.

3. Decide that you really need the increased range of joint motion and the ability to move more freely. Sometimes surgery is the best way to achieve the most dramatic change.

4. Agree with your professional health adviser that you need better alignment of deformed joints. Joints deformed by osteoarthritis, such as in the hip or severely bowed legs from knee joint degeneration, may be ''unlocked'' by surgery, improving the range of motion and relieving pain. The appearance of the joints may improve significantly, although they will probably not be as perfectly aligned as they were before the onset of osteoarthritis.

Before deciding you should also consider the consequences. There are disadvantages to all surgical procedures. These disadvantages fall into three primary categories.

Side Effects

Side effects are unintended peripheral or secondary effects, which may or may not be harmful. They are often temporary discomforts with no lasting negative effects on the body. For example, you may experience some nausea after taking a narcotic pain reliever like codeine; or you may have some loss of sensation on the skin where an incision was made.

Adverse Reactions

More serious than side effects, these can result in permanent harm. For instance, someone with a severe allergy to an anesthetic agent may suffer a life-threatening allergic reaction; or a piece of grafted tissue might be rejected by the recipient's body. Taking NSAIDs for long periods to deal with postoperative pain can lead to kidney damage, which is another example of an adverse drug reaction.

Complications

Complications that lead to some residual impairment are the most feared result of surgery. Examples include a joint infection leading to a joint that does not move much due to excessive scar tissue (arthrofibrosis), or, in the extreme, a heart attack or stroke during surgery.

Failed Outcome

Side effects, adverse reactions, and complications must be distinguished from *failed outcomes*. Too often the surgeon does not emphasize the definition of this term prior to performing the procedure. Failed outcome simply refers to the situation where the procedure did not improve the problem (and may even have worsened it slightly) despite the fact that the procedure was performed correctly and there was no identifiable reason for the failure.

An example of a failed outcome is having an arthritis surgery that does not lessen your pain or improve your range of motion. A more common situation is an injection of cortisone that does not result in any difference in pain or swelling.

Many malpractice lawsuits are the result of poor patient-doctor communication. Sometimes, however, this is not because the doctor was rushed or the patient didn't ask the right questions. Rather, physicians often prefer not to go through the laundry list of potential side effects, adverse reactions, and complications because of the *nocebo* effect. The placebo effect describes the phenomenon where the positive power of suggestion results in an improvement in about 30 percent of people, even if the treatment has no physical reason for working. The nocebo effect works in the same way. Surgeons warning patients to expect side effects or adverse reaction can often "induce" patients to experience those problems. If a doctor explains, "Mrs. Jones, you may have a lot of soreness, nausea, and light-headedness after this injection," there is a good chance that Mrs. Jones will experience all three.

We should hasten to add that the nocebo effect is not an indication that the patient is particularly suggestible or in any way a hysteric. Almost all of us are subject to the power of suggestion, positive and negative. When we are warned about something, we cannot help thinking about it. And thinking often makes it so. (One folktale tells us that you can reach the pot of gold at the end of the rainbow if you are able to walk for an hour through a forest without ever once thinking of an elephant. Tradition has it that no one told of this test has ever managed to pass it!)

Injectables

Before deciding on a more invasive surgical procedure, you should know more about the various injectables now available. Here are several major types of injectable; these can help even intractable cases of osteoarthritis. They often help alleviate the symptoms of rheumatoid arthritis, as well.

Glucocorticoids (cortisone and related steroids)
Glucocorticoids are the prototypical and original anti-inflammatory medications, popular since the 1940s. Cortisone is probably the best known of these medications, but there are many of them available for injections. They are technically *steroids,* i.e., a group of hormones produced naturally in the adrenal cortex and important for the metabolism of carbohydrates and protein. In synthetic form they are highly effective at controlling inflammation. While they are steroids, don't confuse them with androgenic steroids (male hormones like testosterone), which are something else again.

Some glucocorticoids are longer acting with slower onset; others are shorter acting with a quicker onset of symptom relief. Besides this difference, however, physician familiarity is usually the reason for the choice of one product versus another. The most frequently used products are:

- hydrocortisone acetate, which is short acting
- Methylprednisolone acetate, prednisolone sodium phosphate, tebutate, triamcinolone acetonide, diacetate, or hexacetonide, which are all intermediate acting
- Betamethasone acetate, dexamethasone acetate or sodium phosphate, which are long acting

When injected, glucocorticoids stabilize the lysozymes located inside the cell membranes. These lysozymes are chemical-containing packets that tend to inflame and degrade cartilage and its supporting structures in the joint. By stabilizing the lysozymes, the chemicals within them are prevented from being released and causing inflammation.

At the same time, new evidence suggests that glucocorticoids also work by increasing the production of a specific inhibitor protein that blocks *cytokines,* another class of chemicals responsible for inflammation.

BENEFITS AND RISKS

Glucocorticoid injections can keep patients pain-free for weeks or sometimes months at a time. They are therefore useful when trying to delay an arthritis surgery such as a joint replacement, or occasionally, when waiting for your chondroitin/glucosamine treatment to become effective.

Unfortunately, they can cause long-term damage to the cartilage with repeated use. Professional football players were the first to make us aware of the negative impact of injecting glucocorticoids. Many players, especially during the 1960s and 1970s, were repeatedly injected in order to stay in the game. Many later suffered from crippling arthritis as a result. Therefore, patients should realize that, once they start using injected glucocorticoids once or twice per year in the same joint, an eventual joint replacement is almost certain. However, again there is good news—it is now clear that these injections generally prove to be unnecessary. Dr. Theodosakis's clinical use of injected glucocorticoids has fallen to near zero since he started using the treatments earlier recommended in *The Arthritis Cure.*

Sodium Hyaluronate or Hyaluronate

This injectable shows great promise. When injected into the joints, most commonly the knee, its thick viscosity provides lubrication between the synovial membrane and the cartilage and adds to the shock-absorbing ability of the cartilage. Injectable hyaluronic acid replaces the body's own hyaluronic acid that is lost when a joint is affected by osteoarthritis.

In 1993, a state-of-the-art review article analyzed all the then-known studies, many of which were carefully placebo-controlled and very persuasive. Indeed, the improvements were so substantial that the author was able to conclude, "local treatment of osteoarthritis with hyaluronate has already proved to be a valuable and innocuous form of therapy. New developments . . . should help bring a useful relief to osteoarthritic patients for protracted periods, and substantiate the hope of influencing the natural course of this disease."[1] Later, in an editorial for the Osteoarthritis Research Society,[2] Peyron went farther and stated flatly that, "The fact that clinical improvement is sustained and that synovial fluid returns towards normal long after the injected material has left the joint, suggests a lasting influence on the pathophysiological processes of osteoarthritis."

Since that time, many additional research studies have been undertaken, including some not yet published. We anticipate that the preliminary favorable studies mentioned above will largely be confirmed once the new articles have been subjected to careful peer review.

1. Jacques Peyron, "Inarticular Hyaluronan Injections in the Treatment of Osteoarthritis," *Journal of Rheumatology* 20, no. 39 (1993): 10–15.
2. Jacques Peyron, editorial, *Osteoarthritis and Cartilage* 1 (1993): 85–87.

BENEFITS AND RISKS

The product was approved for use in the United States only in the summer of 1997, so physicians here are still gaining experience in its use. However, it has been widely used in other countries since 1987 (there have been more than 1.5 million patient uses), and a large number of clinical studies have shown that, correctly injected, hyaluronic acid can reduce pain and improve mobility. Its effectiveness compares well to the NSAIDs in terms of pain relief but with the huge advantage of not being associated with the potentially harmful side effects and drug interactions of the NSAIDs. More important, hyaluronic acid is being studied to assess its possible benefit in preventing arthritis progression.

Hyaluronic acid injections are given directly into the joint with a tiny needle after the skin has been numbed with lidocaine. The procedure is no more uncomfortable than having blood drawn, and certainly nowhere near as painful as regular surgery. Moreover, while all injections should be treated with care, these have been well tolerated in clinical studies, and no significant side effects have been noted. Their main disadvantage is that they have to be injected at least three, and up to five, times in order to be fully effective. The cost of the medicine and physician-administered injections is in the $1,000 range. Fortunately, since hyaluronic acid products are FDA-approved, insurance plans are likely to pay part or all of the cost of this therapy.

Proliferative Agents (Dextrose, Hypertonic Saline)

An area that holds great promise in treating many musculoskeletal problems including arthritis is *prolotherapy*. This involves the injection of sterile materials usually into soft tissue such as ligaments, but also occasionally into joints. It provides a nonsurgical method of tightening and healing supportive structures that have been damaged or loosened but not completely torn.

Prolotherapy is also being used in osteoarthritic joints to stimulate the proliferation of fibroblasts (connective-tissue-producing cells) and chondrocytes (cartilage-producing cells). This is a process that can actually lead to improvement in the health of joint tissues. Although evidence is still limited, some clinicians also believe that prolotherapy may have a slight *neurolytic* effect, that is, it may decrease or eliminate the painful sensation transmitted by the small nerve fibers contained within ligamentous or connective tissue structures.

BENEFITS AND RISKS

In the best case, prolotherapy can relieve pain in those cases that have not responded well to medication, physical therapy, or surgery. It can be used for a variety of conditions, such as chronic pain in the lower back, neck, and structures outside and around joints. Sometimes, when minor laxity exists, prolotherapy can provide enough joint stabilization to preclude the need for reconstructive surgery. Prolotherapy thus provides another valuable tool for treating a variety of problems that may directly or indirectly affect the overall condition of the musculoskeletal system.

Since prolotherapy usually involves a series of injections, the risk of infection is a concern. In addition, there is a lack of long-term outcome studies. However, this is also true for most of the procedures prolotherapy is designed to replace.

The Risks of Injectables

Injectable medications are considered to be the least invasive of the surgical procedures for treating osteoarthritis. The general risks of any injection are bleeding, infection, and adverse reactions to the medication. If the needle used in the injection penetrates an artery or vein, excessive bleeding can occur, especially with patients who are taking a blood thinner like Coumadin (warfarin) or even aspirin. However, it is very rare that this bleeding cannot be stopped or leads to long-term problems.

An infection in a joint is a somewhat bigger concern. Joint injections carry a higher risk of infection than ordinary injections because the inside of joints do not have good blood flow to supply bacteria-eating white blood cells. Moreover, if the joint has been operated on previously, especially if it contains screws of other artificial parts, the risk of infection increases. Any bacteria accidentally introduced into the joint space become attached to the artificial parts and multiply rapidly. In that case, IV antibiotics and surgery to remove the artificial parts may become necessary.

The last main category of risks due to injections relates to the medication introduced into the joint. A small percentage of people given a cortisone injection experience a loss of skin pigmentation if the medicine seeps up to the skin's surface. And, in rare cases, emotional irritability or extreme agitation results from the medication.

Nevertheless, although there are some potential risks from injections, they are slight, and injectables can help bridge the gap between oral medications such as glucosamine and chondroitin and surgery.

Surgeries

We hope and expect that, for many of you, the full application of our program, including the enhancements noted in this book, will make surgery unnecessary. If not, your first fallback position should be the injectables noted above, which, together with our program, should resolve the problem. However, if your osteoarthritis is already so advanced that even this is not enough and surgery is required, the first thing you owe yourself is to be fully informed. That is the purpose of the rest of this chapter.

In the "old days," back before the 1960s, there wasn't much that surgery could do for osteoarthritis. The best approach was to smooth out the irregular joint surfaces, but often that wasn't terribly helpful. Sometimes the surgeon simply fused the affected joint, which initially took care of the pain but often led to other problems as patients had to compensate for the loss of motion in the fused joint. (Have you ever tried to walk with your knee locked?)

Fortunately, surgeries for arthritic joints have improved dramatically. For example, where it is appropriate, arthroscopic surgery is much less traumatic than the older approaches. In this procedure, the surgeon makes three small incisions in the skin near a joint. A small fiber-optic instrument is inserted through one of the holes, surgical instruments through another, while the third hole serves as an irrigation port for sterile salt-water that cleans and enlarges the joint. The surgeon can take stock of the situation by looking through the arthroscope, or by watching a small screen to which the instrument is attached. Special instruments can then be inserted through the arthroscope into the joint to remove pieces of free-floating cartilage or bone fragments that are "jamming" the joint. Since there is very little blood loss or tissue damage, recovery time is much shorter with arthroscopy than with the older forms of surgery.

Here are some of the many joint surgeries used to relieve the symptoms of osteoarthritis. They are listed from the least to the most invasive.

Arthroscopic Washout or Lavage

The simplest and least invasive surgical procedure is an arthroscopic washout or lavage which is usually performed under general anesthesia or a spinal. Sometimes, a surgeon does arthroscopic surgery for diagnostic reasons. Since the procedure involves flushing the joint with large amounts of sterile saline, loose debris in the joint is removed along with a temporary reduction in some of the enzymes that break down the damaged cartilage. No drilling or cutting instruments are used other than blunt probes to look at the various parts of the knee. Some patients do quite well after this procedure for periods of up to a year. Diagnostic arthroscopies are being performed less and less, however, because many insurance companies won't cover a procedure that has not been deemed "definitive."

Scar Tissue Release

After a previous surgery or injury, excessive scar tissue may form around a joint and lead to increased pressure on some of the cartilage surfaces. For example, the kneecap often develops a band of scarring that causes one side of it to rub on the cartilage, wearing it down and leading to osteoarthritis. Joint malalignment is one of the well-known contributing factors to osteoarthritis, which can occur not only in the knee but also in fingers, elbows, and shoulders. Typically, a patient may be doing well after surgery only to find a worsening of the symptoms many months or even years later as the scar tissue affects the joint. Fortunately, correcting the problem usually involves some minor trimming of the scar tissue to free up the affected area, followed by some physical therapy and tissue massage.

Joint Surface Debridement

Developed in 1946, this procedure is used to smooth irregular joint surfaces either by removing loose fragments of cartilage, osteophytes (bone spurs), or an overgrown synovium (joint lining), and/or by shaving areas on the surface of the cartilage in order to prevent locking or catching of the joint. After the surface has been smoothed, the joint is irrigated with large quantities of fluid.[3] One of the main goals of debridement is to get the joint to fill in the worn-down cartilage with scar tissue. This scar tissue, called fibrocartilage, does not have the same low-friction or shock absorption properties as the original articular cartilage, but it does help decrease the amount of bone overgrowth that would occur with simply leaving the bony surface exposed.

For the best possible results after a debridement, the joint should have had an adequate range of motion and have been in alignment. The patient must also do postsurgical exercises to restore mobility lost through surgery. Recovery time can be six to twelve months. To help with the recovery, a rehabilitation technique called *continuous passive motion* or CPM is

3. K. E. Kuetter and W. M. Goldberg, "Osteoarthritic Disorders," American Academy of Orthopaedic Surgeons symposium, 1995.

often used.[4] As the name implies, CPM keeps the joints moving slowly but continually while the patient is in a passive position (for example, lying down or even sleeping). In other words, a machine does all the work while the patient rests. This increases the range of motion and keeps the joint from stiffening. CPM has also been shown to help cartilage grow better after surgery. Depending on the circumstances, a patient may use CPM for up to eight hours per day for eight or more weeks.

Besides relieving pain, debridement is supposed to result in a smooth surface and was believed to help slow the progression of osteoarthritis. However, the fibrocartilage scar that forms from the procedure usually breaks down in a few years (or sometimes even in months), so researchers are not sure whether this procedure actually results in better long-term outcomes. Most people feel better for six to twenty-four months, although 10–15 percent actually feel more pain after the procedure. Debridement surgery is performed primarily on the knee, and sometimes on the ankle, wrist, or elbow.

Debridement is still used by most orthopedic surgeons as the standard care for osteoarthritis that is not severe enough to warrant a joint replacement. However, its days are probably numbered as more promising procedures become available.

Cartilage/Bone Grafts

In this procedure, cartilage, usually connected to a plug of bone, is grafted onto a hole drilled in the affected joint. The graft is sized to fit perfectly within the drilled hole. The donor bone (with the attached cartilage) eventually becomes enmeshed with the patient's own bone, just as occurs with any bone graft. Cartilage alone is not used in a graft because it is too soft to be secured to the underlying bone. Donor bone with attached cartilage can be taken from a non-weight-bearing

4. Steadman, J. Richard et al., "Improvement of Full-Thickness Chondral Defect Healing in the Human Knee After Debridement and Microfracture Using Continuous Passive Motion," *American Journal of Knee Surgery* 7, no. 3 (Summer 1994): 109–16.

surface in the same patient, or from a cadaver.

An earlier concern with transplanting tissue from others was the risk of life-threatening infections such as HIV or hepatitis. However, although some risk still remains, with today's newer methods of analyzing tissue, it is low.

Cartilage grafts work best in patients with specific, isolated areas of degenerated joint cartilage, and some studies have shown that they can delay or even prevent further degeneration.[5] But these grafts have generally been used in salvage operations after major trauma (such as an automobile accident), and usually in patients under the age of forty. Cartilage grafts do not seem to work well on those with osteoarthritis. However, more work is being done in this area.

Osteotomy

Osteo is Greek for "bone," and *tomy* means "cutting," so an osteotomy is a cutting of the bone.

Picture the Leaning Tower of Pisa. If you were able to cut a wedge out of the base of the "high" side and affix the cut to the bottom of the "low" side, the tower's name would have to be changed. This is essentially what is done in an osteotomy.

One of the earliest forms of surgery for osteoarthritis, osteotomy is designed to realign the bones and redirect the pressure to a less worn-out area of joint surface. This is accomplished by cutting the bone, realigning it, and thus redistributing the force exerted on the joint. Then the worn-out cartilage, now relieved of grinding pressure, can repair and restore itself. Taking glucosamine and chondroitin sulfates well before this surgery gives the cartilage a significant head start on the road to recovery. And continuing the therapy after surgery helps the cartilage to continue healing.

Osteotomy is usually performed on the knees of patients under the age of sixty who have many years to live and might

5. R. C. Locht et al., "Late Osteochondral Allograft Resurfacing for Tibial Plateau Fractures," *Journal of Bone and Joint Surgery* 66-A (March 1984): 328–35.

"wear out" a joint replacement, thus requiring a second one. (Second joint replacements are much riskier than first replacements and don't last as long, so surgeons prefer to perform initial replacements on older people.) Osteotomies are also considered when one area of a patient's joint is ailing but another area is still good. For example, if the inside compartment of the knee has lost quite a bit of cartilage, but the lateral side is still good, osteotomy may be performed so that you don't have to discard the good side by replacing the entire joint.

Osteotomies can lead to dramatic pain relief, greatly enhanced joint function, and improved joint motion and stability. But the surgery works best on patients who still have some range of motion prior to surgery, who meet certain criteria for joint alignment, and who will be able to follow an intensive postoperative exercise plan. Otherwise, they may lose some joint function.

Some patients remain satisfied for as long as twenty years after they have had osteotomies, but most patients experience benefits for only a few years. This is an important consideration, because the altered joint alignment from an osteotomy can occasionally make later joint replacement more difficult.

Joint Replacement

In this surgery, technically called *joint arthroplasty,* an entire joint is removed and replaced by an artificial joint made of metal, plastic, or a ceramic material. Joint replacement, a well-established technique, is usually performed on the hip and knee joints, although recently it has also been successful on shoulders, elbows, ankles, and knuckles.

The number of these procedures performed in the United States exceeds 500,000 per year, including 120,000 hips[6] and

6. NIH Consensus Conference, *Journal of the American Medical Association* 273, no. 24 (June 28, 1995): 1950–56.

95,000 knees.[7] The results are generally best for the hip, followed by the knee and the other joints, probably because the hip joint has a less complicated structure and function.

During replacement of the hip, a ball-and-socket structure, the femoral head ("ball") of the arthritic bone is first removed. A metal stem with a metal ball attached is then cemented into the hollow portion of the femur where the old femur head used to be. A plastic socket, held in place by cement, is used to line the arthritic hip socket. The metal or ceramic ball can then glide smoothly within its new plastic socket, creating very little friction. Destruction of the hip, a centrally located joint, can be extremely debilitating, so successful replacement can be of huge benefit.

Total joint replacement is successful in the sense that it goes according to plan about 96 percent of the time.[8] Of course, the new joint doesn't compare to the patient's original one in stability and function. Still, the pain relief and improved function can give the patient a new lease on life.

There can be serious complications from this operation. The most common is that, over time, the cement holding the socket lining in place can crack and break into little fragments, allowing the implant to loosen. When the body attempts to remove these cement fragments, it can also remove bits of the bone to which they are attached, weakening its overall structure. You can reduce your chances of suffering from a "loose implant" by choosing a surgeon experienced in joint replacement, avoiding high-stress activities such as running and heavy weight lifting, keeping your body weight at an acceptable level, and taking steps to keep your bones from losing minerals and becoming osteoporotic.

Cementless hip replacements are now used in many cases to avoid loosening of the prosthesis. The cementless parts have

7. M. Brittberg, "Treatment of Deep Cartilage Defects in the Knee with Autologous Chondrocyte Transplantation," *New England Journal of Medicine* 331, no. 14 (October 6, 1994): 889–95.

8. H. D. Huddleston, *Arthritis of the Hip Joint*, 3rd ed. 1995, p. 26–28.

a very bumpy, porous surface that resembles coral growing on a reef. The bone actually grows into this rough surface, anchoring it in place naturally. Unfortunately, the bones of some older patients and patients with soft bones or osteoporosis may not be able to bond well with this kind of prosthesis. But those under the age of sixty who have normal bones are usually advised to use cementless hip replacements.

The main concern about joint replacement, aside from the fact that it is a major operation, is the life span of the replacements, which average about ten to fifteen years for hips and eight to twelve years for knees. While technology and surgeons' knowledge keeps improving, not all insurance plans pay for newer procedures. Therefore, be sure to discuss this issue with your surgeon if you are considering joint replacement.

Invasive Treatments for Joint Laxity/Joint Instability

Not all surgeries and injections for arthritis are performed on the joint cartilage. For example, it is well known that a joint dislocation or subluxation (near-dislocation) can eventually lead to osteoarthritis, possibly because the excessive "play" in the joint tips the balance of the normal cartilage breakdown/cartilage buildup equation further toward degeneration. Injections, such as prolotherapy (described earlier), can help stabilize such joints to a small degree, but surgery is often necessary. For example, a skier who tears the anterior cruciate ligament in his or her knee is less likely to develop osteoarthritis later by undergoing a ligament reconstruction procedure to "tighten" up the joint now. This procedure involves stabilizing the knee by affixing a ligament or tendon, either from a cadaver or from another area of the patient's own body, into approximately the same location as the site of the original ligament. Of course, a long course of rehabilitation to regain strength, coupled with proper biomechanics, is essential to the outcome of this procedure.

Ligament reconstruction has become a common procedure, performed well by hundreds of competent orthopedic surgeons on spines, shoulders, elbows, wrists, fingers, and ankles.

Microfracture

This new surgical procedure is worth bringing to your attention because it may prove to have immense value in the future.

Microfracture, a surgical technique pioneered by Dr. Richard Steadman of Vail, Colorado, is a refinement of what is called subchondral bone penetration. During microfracture surgery, a special surgical awl that functions like an ice pick is used to poke tiny holes in the bone beneath the damaged area of the cartilage.

Unlike skin and other body tissues, which easily form scar tissue, cartilage does not repair itself well. This is partly because it lacks its own blood vessels and must rely on the relatively inefficient mechanism of synovial fluid washing back and forth to bring in nutrients and healing factors and carry away waste products. With microfracture, however, nutrients and healing growth factors from the bone marrow are able to reach the newly exposed healthy cartilage. A blood clot forms, and the healing process begins. Dr. Steadman believes that the blood clot contains marrow-derived pluripotential stem cells that have the ability to mature into other types of cells, including chondrocytes, which may encourage the growth of new cartilage.

Used on more than one thousand patients since the mid-1980s, microfracture has shown a great deal of promise. The surgery helped Hilary Lindh, an Olympic silver medalist who won gold in the 1997 world skiing championships after undergoing microfracture surgery. And Bruce Smith, defensive end for the Buffalo Bills, was voted the National Football League's Defense Player of the Year in 1996 after having the surgery on both knees. When combined with CPM—continuous passive movement—the new cartilage may last for years.

However, the surgery is not always successful, with several factors contributing to a bad outcome, including severe joint degeneration, bad joint alignment, certain patterns of joint use, and the patient's age. Even if the surgery is successful, the new cartilage may lack some of the properties that allow normal, healthy cartilage to withstand and effectively distribute pressure.

Nevertheless, we suspect that microfracture will eventually replace debridement as one of the mainstays of arthritis surgery, especially if the procedure is combined with the use of glucosamine and chondroitin pre- and postoperatively.

Autologous Chondrocyte Implantation

The concept behind this surgery, known as ACI, is to harvest healthy cartilage cells from cartilage a little distance away from the damaged area of the joint and use them to regrow the damaged cartilage. The procedure is to prepare the harvested cells carefully, and then place them into a solution of culture medium and fluid (serum) extracted from the patient's own body, where they can continue to grow and multiply. After a few weeks, these healthy cartilage cells are then injected into the damaged area of the joint where they continue to grow into healthy cartilage.

ACI is being used in cartilage defects due to trauma (a form of secondary osteoarthritis). We know that trauma-induced osteoarthritis occurs following a direct insult to the chondrocytes. A severe impact or blow to the articular cartilage, for instance, causes the chondrocytes to slow their production of collagen and proteoglycans, and increase their production of cartilage-destroying enzymes. This results in the breakdown of the articular structure that is the hallmark of osteoarthritis. The theory behind using ACI in these cases is to replace the damaged, cartilage-destroying chondrocytes with healthy new ones, thus restoring the balance to the cartilage metabolism.

The long-term durability of the regenerated cartilage is not yet known since this procedure is relatively new. There is some speculation that the success of the procedure may be significantly enhanced by rapidly transplanting the cultured chondrocytes into the cartilage defect. This can be done by culturing the cells in a location near the operating suite, thus avoiding the delay in having the cells sent via the mail. As with any transplanted tissue or organ, the time from harvesting to implantation directly impacts success or failure.

Early results with ACI are promising. However, the surgery is best suited for people under the age of forty who have suffered a traumatic injury resulting in a single lesion of the femur (one of the two bones in the lower leg). The whole procedure, including the special cell culturing, costs as much as $40,000. Understandably, therefore, health insurance companies have balked at approving this procedure until there are better long-term outcome studies.

The Risks of Surgery

There's no doubt that surgery can work wonders, but it is risky.

How can you tell which surgeries are likely to be dangerous? Follow this general rule: Any big surgery is risky, and any surgery done on you is big! Anytime you undergo anesthesia while someone cuts into your skin, muscles, tendons, ligaments, and/or bones, you run the risk of infection, nerve damage, blood clots, and more. Other potential drawbacks of surgery include:

- *Discomfort*   The body doesn't like being sliced into with a knife, having pieces of it cut apart, trimmed, rearranged, and sewn together. Postsurgical discomfort, ranging from mild to almost unbearable, is all but inevitable. And if you have surgery on weight-bearing joints such as the knees or hips, you may continue to feel quite a bit of pain for a lengthy period because these joints have to support large amounts of weight when you move around.
- *Infection*   Cutting into the body gives bacteria an easy entry. The overall risk is relatively small because modern surgical techniques are good, but even a small infection can cloud the outcome of the surgery. The chances of infection are increased with conditions such as diabetes, or behaviors such as smoking.
- *Blood clots*   There is a small risk of developing a blood clot after surgery. The clot can "stick" where it forms, clogging a blood vessel and stopping the flow of blood. Or it may drift through the bloodstream after forming, clogging a

vessel elsewhere. The type and extent of damage caused by the clot both depend on where it sticks. If it happens in the lungs, it can cause a pulmonary embolism that destroys part of the lungs. Clots in the arterial system are less common but can be deadly. Clots lodging in the brain or heart can trigger strokes and heart attacks, respectively. These risks are all tiny statistically, but they exist and you should be aware of them.

- *Dangerous decline in fitness*   Especially in older people, even brief periods of surgery-induced immobility may lead to a severe loss of fitness. People who are unfit to begin with may find themselves too weak even to walk to the bathroom. One of the best ways to prevent a decline in fitness after surgery is to start physical therapy *before* having the surgery, because the prognosis of any joint surgery is improved by presurgical therapy. Your insurance company may balk, but this is the one time you may consider paying for a few sessions yourself. Additionally, patients should undergo plenty of physical therapy starting almost immediately following surgery.

- *Adverse effect from anesthesia*   There is also the very small possibility of complications from anesthesia. Of course, older people and those with severe health problems are at greater risk here.

Who Should Perform Your Surgery?
If, after much deliberation, you decide to have surgery, selecting a surgeon may be the most important decision you ever make.

Your regular doctor may be your most appropriate referral source. But remember, doctors have been known to refer their buddies in order to give them business, and many doctors are now forced by their health maintenance organizations (HMOs) to suggest surgeons on their HMO's list.

Therefore, in addition to seeking your own doctor's advice, you can call your local hospital, medical center, or medical society for referrals, and you can look through *The Best Doc-*

tors in America, published annually. No doubt, you will want to ask your acquaintances who have had the kind of surgery that you're considering for opinions of their own surgeons. But remember, they may not have checked as carefully as you would, and a single positive outcome means little. Even the worst surgeons have many successes, and the best have occasional failures. It is the *percentage* of success that is important.

Sometimes this information is available for a whole category of surgery you are contemplating. In that case, you can ask the surgeon for his or her outcome statistics and compare. If the data are not available, though, it is often a good idea to ask several good surgeons whom they would hire if they were having that particular procedure done on themselves. Another good trick is to go to a busy physical therapy office and ask the therapists which doctor's patients seem to do the best after surgery.

Teaching hospitals are often full of well-qualified, knowledgeable surgeons who are up-to-date on current procedures and practices. But keep in mind that July is the month when most new trainees start their residencies (and are, thus, at their least experienced). The attending physician at the teaching hospital is responsible for overseeing the actions of the trainees, but not all attending physicians are able to properly supervise every step or phase of every single surgery. On the other hand, you sometimes actually get more attentive care at teaching hospitals, from both the young surgeons and their supervisor. The important point is to find out who will be doing the surgery on you and who will be supervising. Will they both be in the operating theater while you are in surgery?

Most important of all, make sure your surgeon has had extensive experience in performing the exact surgery that you are considering. Ask for references from past patients who are willing to talk about their experience. Then call them to learn all you can about both the surgery, its aftermath, and the surgeon.

Interviewing Potential Surgeons

You can—and should—interview the doctor who wants to operate on you, just as you would question anyone before offering him or her a job. Once you've identified several well-qualified, highly recommended candidates, schedule appointments to interview them. Come prepared with questions (such as those below) and take charge of the interview.

Have the surgeon explain the procedure to you in detail, politely insisting that all of your questions be answered completely. Don't be shy about asking for information. It's your body. You're the one taking the risks, *you're* the one who will be living with the results. And you're footing the bill! If the surgeon seems reluctant to speak to you, or is curt or unpleasant, look for another. And always get a second, even a third, opinion whenever you're considering surgery—not because you don't trust the doctor, but because different doctors often have differing opinions as to the best surgical approach. (Disqualify a surgeon who balks when you say you'd like to get another opinion.)

Knowledge is power. The more you know, the better decisions you can make. And you may find out that you don't need the surgery after all. Here are some good questions to ask the surgeons whom you interview.

- Exactly what happens during the surgery you are recommending?
- How long does the procedure take?
- Describe all the side effects, from the most to the least likely.
- What patients are most likely to suffer these side effects? What are my risks of having them?
- How much blood am I likely to lose during the surgery?
- Will I need a transfusion? Can I stockpile some of my own blood to be used?
- Will you be transplanting tissue to me in any manner? If so, how is this tissue screened for diseases like hepatitis or HIV?
- How much pain will I experience after the surgery? And for how long?

- How will my pain be managed?
- Will I have a scar? If so, where will it be, how long and thick will it be? Can you do anything to lessen the scar? Can the scar be "fixed" with plastic surgery later?
- What kind of anesthesia will be used? What are the effects of the anesthesia?
- What is the anesthetist's name? Will I be able to meet with the anesthetist before the surgery and have my questions answered?
- Who will actually perform the surgery, you or one of your associates? Will trainees be working on me as well?
- How often is this surgery successful overall? How often when you perform it?
- How many of these surgeries have you performed? Over what period of time?
- Are you board certified in orthopedics? Did you take a fellowship in any particular surgical subspecialty?
- Where will the surgery be performed?
- How do the infection rates compare between this hospital and others in the area?
- Should I stop taking any of my medications before the surgery? Which ones, and how soon before?
- Will I need any medications after surgery? Which ones, why, and for how long?
- Should I have any physical therapy before surgery? (We recommend this, even if you have to pay for it yourself.)
- Will I need physical therapy or have to perform exercises after surgery?
- How long before I'm up and around, able to take care of myself, and able to return to work? How long before I can move my joint normally?
- Why do you favor the surgery you are recommending over another? What other surgeries might be used?
- Do you have informational material I can study?

Ask these questions, plus any others you think are important. Nothing is too small or insignificant to bring up. To have or not to have a surgical procedure is one of the most important decisions you will ever make.

And remember: *You are not required to allow any doctor to operate on you just because you've interviewed him or her, or because you've signed a consent form. You are free to change your mind at any time, for any reason, right up to the moment before the anesthesiologist puts you to sleep.*

Prior to Surgery

If you decide to have surgery, your preparations should begin at least a couple weeks before the surgery date. You will undoubtedly be asked to undergo a battery of medical tests to ensure that you are healthy enough to withstand the surgery. If you need to and are able to donate your own blood, do so well in advance of the surgery in order to give your body plenty of time to recover. Your surgeon will give you the specifics on preparation, but you should be aware of the following standard presurgical steps:

- If you smoke, try to stop as far ahead of your surgery as you can.
- Take extra care to eat a balanced diet. Ask your doctor if you need to supplement your diet with any vitamins, minerals, or other substances.
- Your surgeon will tell you if and when to discontinue your medications prior to surgery. Some drugs, such as aspirin, can be dangerous to those undergoing surgery because they can lead to excessive bleeding. However, generally, subject to checking with your surgeon, you should continue taking chondroitin/glucosamine right up to your surgery and start again immediately following it. In most cases, this improves the surgical outcome and speed of recovery.
- Be sure to plan ahead to ensure that your job, household, pets, or other responsibilities are taken care of so that you don't need to worry or have any crises while you are recovering.
- If you need splints, a cane, or a wheelchair, make sure you have them in advance.

- Get any existing infections (including genitourinary, vaginal, and skin) treated before the surgery.
- See your dentist to get any cavities filled or oral infections treated, lest these infections spread once you undergo the stress of surgery.

The Recovery Period

Once surgery is over, you have only one thing in mind: getting better as soon as possible. With most surgeries on a joint in your hand or arm, you'll probably be up and around the day of the surgery. If you have surgery on weight-bearing joints, such as the hip, knee, or ankle, you may be confined to bed or to a chair for a week or longer (though the trend is to try to get most people "up" as early as possible). Your doctor will let you know when it's safe to get up and begin moving around with the aid of a walker, crutches, or a walking cast.

Pain is normal right after surgery and during the first stages of physical therapy. Surprisingly, this pain usually radiates from the muscle rather than from the joint, especially if your muscles were cut into during the surgery. Physical therapy helps relieve this pain while improving joint and muscle function. Working your exercises may be uncomfortable and seem to take forever, but physical therapy does pay off. Conversely, skimping on your physical therapy today causes long-term problems tomorrow.

Finally, let us repeat, don't decide on surgery until you are *sure* the arthritis cure really doesn't work for you. Give it a fair trial. If you do, you may be surprised by how much better you feel. Surgery may turn out to be a needless worry after all.

11

Questions and Answers

After receiving thousands of calls, letters, faxes, and E-mail responses to *The Arthritis Cure,* we couldn't wait to write this chapter. Most of the feedback we received was extremely gratifying, with people reporting that the program was having a tremendous, positive influence. Some people had questions, especially about the supplements. We wish we had the time to respond to each and every person's letter; let this chapter serve as that response. In it, we will answer the questions most commonly asked and give referral information if you need to find out more.

General Questions About the Program

What is the arthritis cure?
Although the supplements called glucosamine and chondroitin have received the lion's share of the attention, the original arthritis cure is actually a nine-point program for dealing with osteoarthritis as outlined in Chapter 2. In this book, we have provided you with a guide to the five principles of maximizing the arthritis cure. To recap, to get the most out of the arthritis cure, you should:

• Involve your physician closely in your care, as outlined in Chapter 3.

- Implement our program of biomechanics described in Chapter 4.
- Follow our exercise program, as outlined in Chapter 5.
- Create a healthful diet for yourself following our nutrition plan, as outlined in Chapter 6.
- Add the specific supplements recommended in Chapter 7 to further enhance healing.

With the help of the arthritis cure, as maximized in this book, we are confident that you can overcome your problem. So we urge you to get started at once, beginning with a trip to your physician.

What does glucosamine do?

Made up of sugar (glucose) and an amino acid, glucosamine is needed for the body to manufacture the proteoglycans that help to keep the cartilage fluid and functional. Glucosamine helps to reduce pain and improve joint function in those afflicted with osteoarthritis. It has also been shown to inhibit at least two of the enzymes that degrade cartilage and has certain *antireactive* properties. This means that glucosamine actually blunts the damaging effects of certain chemicals on the cartilage in joints.

What are chondroitin sulfates?

Chondroitin sulfates are long molecular chains composed of sugar units that help attract fluid into the water-loving proteoglycans. Chondroitin sulfate supplements help diminish the cartilage-destroying enzymes in joints affected by osteoarthritis.

Why is fluid important to cartilage health?

Fluid helps to absorb shock in the joints and carries with it the nutrients cartilage needs to remain healthy. Since cartilage does not have a network of blood vessels to bring in oxygen and nutrients, and carry away waste products, it depends on the steady ebb and flow of fluid for nourishment and cleansing.

What is biomechanics?

Biomechanics is the study of the mechanical forces exerted by and on the body during movement. More practically speaking, biomechanics teaches us ways of standing, sitting, walking, kneeling, lifting, and otherwise moving through the day without placing undue stress on our bodies. Biomechanical techniques and exercises can help reduce osteoarthritis pain by allowing the force from movement to dissipate evenly through the body.

How does exercise help osteoarthritis?

Exercise encourages the flow of cushioning and nourishing fluid into the cartilage. In addition, it strengthens the muscles, tendons, and ligaments that support the joints, which in turn leads to less force being placed on the cartilage during activity. Exercise also increases a joint's range of motion, improves flexibility, and strengthens overall health. Exercise is an excellent ''medicine'' for osteoarthritis.

Why is a good diet important for fighting osteoarthritis?

A healthful diet supplies plenty of the many nutrients the body needs to build strong joints; contains antioxidants to control the dangerous free radicals that may encourage osteoarthritis and other diseases by destroying body tissues; contains bioflavonoids to strengthen joints; contains certain types of fats like EPA and GLA, that may reduce inflammation; and contains zinc, potassium, vitamin C, and other nutrients that counteract some of the harmful effects of commonly prescribed arthritis medications.

How does losing weight help?

Excess weight puts more stress on the osteoarthritis joints of the feet, ankles, knees, hips, and spine. Slimming down to your ideal body weight removes that unnecessary, painful load and thereby helps to prevent osteoarthritis from developing; it also eases the burden should it strike.

How are depression and osteoarthritis linked?

Depression does not cause osteoarthritis, but it makes every-thing—pain, lack of mobility, having to give up various ac-tivities—seem much worse. In fact, many people who develop a chronic pain syndrome find that their pain/disability is made worse by their depression, their depression grows deeper as their pain/disability continues, and they continue spiraling downward. Avoiding depression, and aggressively treating it should it exist, is an important part of your treatment.

If the arthritis cure is so good, why do you recommend the use of "traditional medicines as necessary"?

Although many people respond fairly quickly to glucosamine, chondroitin sulfates, and the rest of the program, some cases are stubborn and take a long time to respond. Some people's joints had been deteriorating for decades before this treatment program was even invented. Traditional treatments, including medications and surgery, may be necessary, especially for those who have little or no cartilage left. Remember, despite the wonders of the arthritis cure treatment program, no single treatment for any disease works on everyone. Even if medi-cations or surgical procedures are required, maximizing the arthritis cure is an important adjunct to making those treat-ments more effective.

If the two books, The Arthritis Cure *and* Maximizing the Arthritis Cure, *spell out the entire program, why must I see a doctor?*

It's important that you begin by seeing a medical doctor to make the proper diagnosis. Other conditions can "masquer-ade" as osteoarthritis and may need very different treatment. Your physician can also monitor your progress, refer you to other appropriate resources as necessary, administer other ther-apies if required, and watch out for treatment reactions and interactions to assist you as you work through the program.

Is the arthritis cure a treatment for rheumatoid or other forms of arthritis?

Although some preliminary evidence suggests that glucosamine and chondroitin sulfates may be of value in treating rheumatoid arthritis, it's too early to say that the two supplements effectively combat rheumatoid arthritis. However, there is no doubt that for patients with both osteo- and rheumatoid arthritis, these supplements can help. Beyond that, many people, including many physicians, are using this program as an adjunct to treating a number of other forms of arthritis.

Is the arthritis cure a treatment for disk disease in the spine or meniscus cartilage injuries in the knee?

There has been some experimental evidence that glucosamine at least has a role in the healing of these cartilaginous tissues. Certainly taking glucosamine and chondroitin sulfates makes theoretical sense in this situation. You should not be too disappointed, however, if you do not experience much effect. These types of cartilage do not have very effective self-repair mechanisms.

Some Specific Questions About Glucosamine and Chondroitin Sulfates

How long does it take for glucosamine and chondroitin to begin working?

Some people notice an effect within a few days, while others may have to wait up to eight weeks. Very rarely, we hear of patients needing three to four months to notice an effect. If there's no noticeable improvement in pain or function after eight to twelve weeks, we advise people to stop using glucosamine and chondroitin sulfates but to continue with the other steps of the arthritis cure.

Can I take glucosamine and chondroitin with anti-inflammatory pills (NSAIDs) or acetaminophen (such as Tylenol)?

Yes, the combinations are safe. In fact, using glucosamine with NSAIDs may be helpful. Some evidence suggests that using glucosamine counteracts the normal decrease in proteoglycan (cartilage) synthesis associated with the use of some NSAIDs. Fortunately, most patients are able to stop using their NSAIDs after taking glucosamine and chondroitin for two to eight weeks. Some who have been taking NSAIDs for decades have been able to get off them completely.

There are many brands on the market. Which do you recommend?

We recommend one of the combination products (containing both glucosamine and chondroitin in one pill or capsule), because people have an easier time sticking to the program when they have to swallow fewer pills. Taking the proper proportions becomes much easier, as well, for the combination products should have glucosamine and chondroitin in the recommended 5:4 ratio in each pill. More important, if you decide to take the products separately (which works just as well if you stick to the regimen), be sure that the products you buy contain the right dosage level, as outlined in *The Arthritis Cure*.

Can I use glucosamine and chondroitin sulfates if I'm allergic to sulfates?

To be safe, patients with sulfate allergies should just take glucosamine *hydrochloride* (not sulfate) and skip the chondroitin sulfate. (We have not found chondroitin in anything but a sulfated form.) Shark cartilage may be a substitute for the chondroitin sulfate, but there's no guarantee that the shark cartilage is not sulfated. And in any case, the amount of the active ingredient you get in shark cartilage is very small. We do not recommend experimenting to see if your sulfate allergy applies to these substances, so you may want to consult with your physician. However, we suspect that this concern is more theoretical than practical. Despite reading many studies and hearing from hundreds of patients taking glucosamine and chondroitin, we have yet to find anyone with a "true" allergic reaction to glucosamine and chondroitin sulfates. (A "true" allergy would produce symptoms such as hives, itching, breathing difficulties, swelling, a drop in blood pressure, passing out, etc.) Still, we assume that there must be some people, somewhere, who are allergic to glucosamine and chondroitin, just as there are people who are allergic to peanuts, strawberries, shellfish, and other common food substances. Be careful if you have, or think you have, any food allergies.

What about food allergies and arthritis?

About 10–15 percent of arthritis sufferers clearly have exacerbations of their arthritis with certain foods. This phenomenon seems to be more common with RA than OA. Studies have shown that fasting for a couple of days can significantly improve RA symptoms in many patients. Some RA patients who become vegetarians tend to feel better, according to an article published in the mainstream journal *Clinical Rheumatology*. Perhaps this diet connection is due to some of the inflammation-promoting substances in meats, such as arachidonic acid.

There has been much debate as to which foods commonly cause arthritis flare-up. Dairy, red meat, shellfish, eggs, yeast, wheat, chocolate, coffee, and nightshade vegetables (eggplant, tomatoes, bell peppers, tobacco, and white potatoes) are the foods most commonly implicated, but some patients report a variety of other foods.

Determining food allergies is often a trial and error affair, so consider eliminating one or more of these foods for a period of a few weeks or months. If you do find a connection, reintroduce the food to see if you notice a worsening of your condition. This confirmation check is wise since many of these foods are healthy in other ways and you would not want to unnecessarily remove them permanently from your diet.

I am pregnant. Should I use glucosamine and chondroitin?

We feel that pregnant women should not take anything except prenatal vitamins unless their physician advises differently. Although there is absolutely no theoretical reason to think that these supplements interfere with pregnancy, there are also no adequate studies to date that have questioned their safety during pregnancy.

I have high blood pressure and take medication. Will glucosamine and chondroitin interact with my medicine or affect my blood pressure?

We are not aware of any known medication interactions with glucosamine and chondroitin. Products containing these supplements, however, often contain some sodium, which can raise blood pressure in people who have salt-sensitive hypertension. This is not a medication interaction but an effect from the sodium itself. We think this reaction to be unlikely, but you should check with your doctor before combining the two.

I have adult-onset diabetes. Will glucosamine and chondroitin raise my blood sugar levels?

We are not aware of any published information on this in humans, nor have we heard of blood sugar elevations in patients taking these supplements. Just to be safe, however, we generally recommend closer monitoring of blood sugar when using these supplements, as well as taking the minimum effective dose. Despite the name similarity, glucosamine and glucose actually have a different pathway of metabolism in the body.

There have been some small studies in rats showing that glucosamine may impair insulin resistance. These studies involve constant intravenous infusions of glucosamine, which is different from intermittent oral dosing. We'd like to see some more human studies in this area.

There are many varieties of glucosamine—what's the difference between them?

The supplement comes in four forms in the United States: glucosamine hydrochloride, glucosamine hydroiodide, n-acetyl glucosamine, and glucosamine sulfate. The sulfate form has the most research evidence to back its use. This is probably because this form was patented in Europe, and more research money was available for its study. Clinically, glucosamine hydrochloride and glucosamine sulfate are identical in terms of their effects. Indeed, the glucosamine hydrochloride form is sulfated in the body anyway. We do not recommend n-acetyl glucosamine, as its action on boosting proteoglycan synthesis is weak, and it doesn't seem to work as well in patients. Glucosamine hydroiodide is not recommended, as the extra iodine may interfere with thyroid function.

Can you use topical glucosamine and chondroitin instead of oral supplements when treating arthritis?

We have not been able to find any information to support the notion that glucosamine and chondroitin are absorbed in any meaningful quantity by topical administration. Theoretical reasoning would tell you that they probably won't. In any case, since the oral forms of these supplements have been shown to be so effective, there's probably no reason to consider another route of entry.

Why hadn't we heard of using glucosamine and chondroitin for arthritis before you published The Arthritis Cure?

The main reason has to do with the Food and Drug Administration's rules. You see, the FDA has ruled that nutritional supplements do not need any government clearance. However, if the manufacturers of such supplements make health claims, then the supplements are deemed to have become "drugs." In that case, before they can be marketed, they have to obtain a "new drug application," which involves huge amounts of testing and often costs more than $100 million. Moreover, with rare exceptions, research conducted outside the United States—even research conducted by highly prestigious universities such as Oxford or Cambridge in England, the University of Tokyo in Japan, the Sorbonne in France, or the leading universities in Germany, Italy, Israel, etc.—is not accepted by the FDA.

Pharmaceutical companies can afford to spend the necessary money on new drug applications if their products are patent-protected so that they can earn back their investment. The problem here is that supplements like those used in the arthritis cure are well known and therefore not patentable. Thus, if some pharmaceutical company were to spend the enormous sum needed to let itself make health claims for a supplement, its competitors would immediately market the same product—and make the same health claims—without having to spend the money to obtain FDA clearance. Consequently, they could afford to sell the product at a lower price.

Naturally, the result of these rules is that major corporations are not very interested in marketing nutritional supplements since they cannot economically justify the expense it would take to make health claims about them, however true those claims may be.

Instead, much smaller companies market the supplements. But they are forced to do so without making any health claims, thus limiting their market. So it is left up to books like this one to provide the correct information about these supplements. Furthermore, it is not so easy to get a book published, and even more difficult to have it reach best-seller status. Therefore, most books, even the ones with highly valuable information, do not become widely known to the general public.

Finally, there is the unfortunate fact that many doctors mistakenly believe that only traditional drugs can be "real medicine." Happily, this situation is changing as more and more physicians—and many teaching hospitals and universities—are recognizing the benefits of alternative and complementary medicine. Soon, we anticipate, complementary remedies like the ones described in this book will become universally recognized. There is even a movement afoot to try to convince the FDA to establish a new category of supplements actually designated as "neutraceuticals" and to allow limited health claims to be made for them without the need for excessive testing and with legitimate overseas research being accepted.

If some is good, why not take more glucosamine and chondroitin?

We have heard stories of people taking 5,000, 6,000, and even 7,000 mg of glucosamine and up to 10,000 mg of chondroitin per day. But we don't believe that this is a good idea. Only chondroitin has been studied in humans at that dosage, and while no harmful side effects were noted, in our opinion, megadoses of almost anything might be harmful. This is true with vitamins and minerals, even water (yes, there is a health condition called "water intoxication"). We therefore recommend that people use the minimum effective dose. High doses don't help the condition more because the body cannot assimilate so much at once, and they could lead to problems of which we are not currently aware.

Questions About Arthritis

Exactly what is osteoarthritis?

Osteoarthritis is the most common form of arthritis. One of over one hundred diseases that can afflict the joints, osteoarthritis involves the articular cartilage, that smooth, glistening, bluish-white substance attached to the ends of bones. Designed to reduce the friction of moving bones rubbing against each other, as well as to absorb some of the shock that comes from movement, this cartilage begins to break down as a result of osteoarthritis. When the protective cartilage weakens, or even disappears, bones can begin to rub against each other. With time, that results in pain, stiffness, joint crackling, bone spurs, abnormal bone hardening, and other problems. Osteoarthritis usually attacks the joints of the knees, hands, hips, feet, and spine. Joints of the shoulders, elbows, wrists, and ankles are less frequent targets.

Is osteoarthritis the "wear-and-tear" type of arthritis?

We used to call osteoarthritis "wear-and-tear" arthritis. Today we distinguish between two types of the disease, primary and secondary. Primary osteoarthritis, the more common type, usually occurs in those forty-five or more years old. A slow, progressive condition, it generally strikes the weight-bearing joints of the hips and knees, as well as the neck, lower back, and fingers. It seems to develop when normal joints are subjected to excessive loads, or normal loads are placed on inferior joints. Exactly why it strikes is not yet known, although it's clear that obesity and family history are contributing factors. The important point is that arthritis is not just an inevitable wearing down of the joints, *caused* by aging.

Secondary arthritis, which can begin in those as young as twenty years old, develops after an injury, joint infection, or other well-defined problem (such as congenital joint malalignment, Paget's disease, and diabetic neuropathy, to name a few).

Are we all destined to get osteoarthritis if we live long enough?

No, although the problem is more common in older than in younger populations. Aged joints may become sore for many reasons, and osteoarthritis is only one of them. Furthermore, less than half of the people who have signs of osteoarthritis have symptoms of pain and limitation from the condition. With osteoarthritis you see deterioration on the weight-bearing surfaces of the cartilage, plus significant changes in the cartilage matrix. Osteoarthritis cartilage and aged normal cartilage differ visibly, biochemically, histologically, and functionally.

Even in the face of a poor family history, there is something you can do to avoid getting osteoarthritis—or suffering from it to any significant degree if you do get it: that is, to follow the plan to maximize the arthritis cure, as described in this book.

What's the difference between osteoarthritis and rheumatoid arthritis?

Rheumatoid arthritis, the second most common form of arthritis, is an autoimmune disease that comes about when the body "turns on itself," attacking body tissue as if it were a dangerous invader. Symptoms of rheumatoid arthritis include discomfort, pain, inflammation, and joint deformity and deterioration. Attacking three times as many women as men, rheumatoid arthritis tends to appear on both sides of the body at once (both wrists, for example).

Why can't I simply take pain pills for my arthritis?

Many people take acetaminophen (Tylenol, Datril, etc.) or nonsteroidal anti-inflammatories (NSAIDs) such as aspirin, Aleve, or MotrinG. These pills successfully block pain and/or inflammation in many cases. However, these medicines (indeed, all medicines) have potentially serious side effects. The NSAIDs, for example, may cause nausea, cramps, diarrhea, ulcers, kidney damage, and even high blood pressure.

It might be worth running the risk of side effects if the standard pain pills actually cured osteoarthritis. But they don't. (In fact, some of them may even worsen the problem.) This means that you're stuck taking the pills forever—and quite likely taking other pills to deal with their side effects. The arthritis cure, on the other hand, can actually eliminate the need to take these medicines altogether, once and for all.

What about the new COX-II inhibitors?

These NSAID variants promise to be a major improvement over the drugs people have been taking for years. With fewer side effects (especially in the gastrointestinal tract), they may be taken for longer periods. They do not cure osteoarthritis, however. And we have not seen reports about the effect of these COX-II inhibitors on cartilage synthesis, so we don't know if they will adversely affect healing as many of the "old" NSAIDs do.

Above all, you should never forget that COX-II inhibitors are still drugs. Thus, they will probably continue to have a variety of interactions with other medications, just as all other NSAIDs do. These drugs may prove to be an important adjunct in the treatment of many forms of arthritis, but they are no cure. The use of chondroitin/glucosamine in conjunction with the rest of the program provided in this book is.

My hip hurts when I push on it. Is that arthritis?
Probably not. If you can cause pain by pushing on the outside of your hip over the area where your hipbone is most prominent, this is most likely bursitis, a condition in which the protective sac, or bursa, is inflamed and painful. Bursae are thin, fluid-filled cushions, usually between a bone and soft tissue, in this case between the greater trochanter and the tensor fascia lata muscle. Due to overuse, injury, or tightness, the muscle rubs firmly on the bone, squishing the bursae, and giving rise to inflammation—pain, swelling, and sometimes warmth. Trochanteric bursitis can last for years and often mimics the symptoms of hip arthritis. Once the bursa is inflamed, it does not heal very easily unless the causative agent is eliminated. An analogy would be biting the inside of your cheek by accident. Once the cheek gets swollen, you continue to bite it and the area does not heal until the biting stops. Trochanteric bursitis is readily curable with specific stretches, such as the Arrow (see page 66), and with the use of cortisone injections.

Other Questions

What do you think of colloidal minerals?
There has been quite a bit of response to an audiotape touting the benefits of various mixtures of "colloidal minerals." Following all mothers' universal advice not to speak if we don't have anything nice to say, we have difficulty responding to

this question. We believe the colloidal mineral marketing fad to be one of the worst ever to come along. Dr. Theodosakis was asked to write a review of all of the "information" contained on the marketing audiotape. After reading four typed pages containing what he believed to be many medical errors, he declined.

Suffice it to say that we know that trace minerals are important. But of the companies selling colloidal products, we have yet to find one—we have asked—willing to provide us with an analysis of what's actually in them. Some of them even list known toxic ingredients on the label! People simply don't need aluminum, lead, arsenic, mercury, or many of the radioactive metals contained in these products. We know of patients who, having used some of these products, experienced hair loss, taste changes, gastrointestinal upset, and other problems.

There is no doubt that trace nutrients are necessary. We advocate a wide variety of fruits and vegetables. "Diet variability" assures that you get all the trace nutrients you need. Taking low doses of other minerals (as mentioned in Chapter 7) is safe and probably helpful.

A Word from Jason Theodosakis, M.D.

All published medical works for the lay press, including the books I have coauthored, are intended for educational purposes only and not meant to offer specific, individual medical advice. I emphasize the need for you to discuss any treatment program, including that put forth in *The Arthritis Cure* and *Maximizing the Arthritis Cure,* with your personal physician.

Although I am a fully accredited physician, a specialist in preventive medicine, and an expert in sports medicine, I am not allowed to answer any of your individual, personal medical, nutrition, referral, or other questions. I may respond only to general questions and general topics. (Indeed, the huge number of requests for more information was the main motivation for writing this follow-up book to *The Arthritis Cure.*)

There are several important reasons why I (or other physicians) cannot respond to personal questions other than from our own patients:

- Any personal or individual advice given would constitute a doctor-patient relationship between us.
- All patient contacts between a doctor and a patient must be charted, and medical records must be kept. This is required by state medical licensing boards. This requirement includes any medical advice given to anyone, no matter how brief or simple the query.
- The hallmark of good diagnosis and treatment is a careful history, physical exam, perhaps X rays, lab work, and other specialized tests. This simply cannot be done over the phone or by letter. Furthermore, following a patient over time and working with other professionals as a team are critical aspects of good care. The best someone could do over the phone would be to get a history, only one part of what's needed for proper care.
- I cannot refer you to another doctor since I would be indirectly liable for that doctor's actions. I cannot guarantee his or her work. I refer only my personal patients to other physicians, doctors whom I know and whose skills I respect.

We hope we have answered all your questions. If you have more, Appendix B provides you with names and addresses of resources you may wish to contact.

In the meantime, though, we urge you to follow the full program outlined in this book. If you do, you will certainly feel much better. And your osteoarthritis may be a thing of the past. The three authors of this book certainly hope so.

Appendix A

New Evidence About the Effectiveness of Chondroitin and Glucosamine

With interest in glucosamine and chondroitin sulfates on the upswing, the results of exciting new studies have recently been presented in medical journals and conferences. For example, several fascinating and persuasive studies were presented at the Third International Congress of the Osteoarthritis Research Society in Singapore, in early June of 1997.[1] What they all boil down to is that the early studies on glucosamine and chondroitin have been confirmed—and expanded! With the ever-increasing data from laboratories and clinics around the world, there's no doubt that glucosamine and chondroitin sulfates have significant benefits for treating osteoarthritis.

In this appendix, we summarize the latest research findings. If you had any doubts about the effectiveness of these supplements before, the new data should eliminate them.

1. Abstracts summarized from *Osteoarthritis and Cartilage*, Vol. 5, Supp. A (Philadelphia: W. B. Saunders, 1997).

Chondroitin Sulfates Help Build New Cartilage[2]

This study was designed to test the ability of chondroitin sulfates to stimulate chondrocytes taken from the joints of human volunteers. Special cells sprinkled throughout the cartilage matrix, chondrocytes are miniature "factories" that manufacture new collagen and proteoglycan molecules. Chondrocytes also produce special enzymes that "chew up" aging collagen and proteoglycan molecules to make room for newer, stronger ones. The activity of these enzymes is termed *collagenolytic activity.*

Chondrocytes were placed in laboratory containers, then mixed with different amounts of chondroitin sulfates (0, 10, 100, and 1,000 μg/ml [millionths of a gram per milliliter]). To see if the chondroitin sulfates had any effect on the chondrocytes, the researchers measured the amount of *new* proteoglycans and type II collagen produced by the chondrocytes, among other things.

Results: Within four to seven days, the chondrocytes mixed with chondroitin sulfate at the two higher doses showed an increase in production of proteoglycans in the chondrocyte clusters. At all three doses of chondroitin sulfate supplementation, a decrease in the collagenolytic activity of the chondrocytes was produced. In other words, chondroitin sulfates are "able to increase proteoglycans in the matrix surrounding the cells" while slowing the destruction caused by "cartilage-eating" enzymes.

2. C. Bassleer and M. Malaise, "Chondroitin Sulfate: Its in Vitro Effect on Human Articular Chondrocytes Cultivated in Clusters."

Chondroitin Sulfates Help Prevent Loss of Knee Cartilage in Rabbits[3]

Researchers from hospitals in Chicago, Illinois, and Geneva, Switzerland, worked together in an effort to determine whether chondroitin sulfates helped the body heal after joint cartilage has been injured.

A special substance (chymopapain) known to damage cartilage was injected into the left knees of twelve rabbits. The animals' right knees served as controls. Some of the animals were also given intramuscular injections or oral doses of chondroitin sulfate (starting ten days before the knee-damaging chymopapain injection and continuing for twenty-one days after).

Eighty-four days later, the animals' knees were examined. The amount of proteoglycans remaining in the knee was used to indicate how much damage had actually occurred.

Results: Examination of the animals who received the cartilage-harming injection but no chondroitin sulfates showed that the cartilage-harming substance chymopapain could reduce the amount of vital proteoglycans down to about 60 percent of normal (normal being the control knees). The reduction of the proteoglycans in the rabbits taking the chondroitin sulfates *orally* was down only to 76 percent of control. The oral-dosing regimen, in fact, bettered the injectable chondroitin in impairing the amount of proteoglycan loss caused by the chymopapain injections. This is evidence of a biologic effect of oral chondroitin on the effect of experimentally induced cartilage loss.

3. D. Uebelhart, J. Zhang, E. J. M. A. Thonar, and J. M. Williams, "Acute Degeneration of Articular Cartilage in the Rabbit: Protective Effect of Chondroitin 4 & 6 Sulfate."

Chondroitin Sulfates Work in Human Knees, Too[4]

The news that chondroitin sulfates work in artifically induced knee cartilage degradation in laboratory animals is exciting. But will it work in humans suffering from real-world osteo-arthritis pain?

Scientists from Hungary's National Institute of Rheumatology and Semmelweis Medical School tested the effects of chondroitin sulfates in a group of patients suffering from osteoarthritis of the knee. This was a powerful, randomized, double-blind, multicenter, placebo-controlled study. The participants were tested at the beginning of the study, as well as at months one, three, and six. All were given either 800 mg of chondroitin sulfates a day or a placebo and were allowed to take as much standard pain medicine (paracetamol) as they wanted. Eighty people completed this double-blind study.

Results: At the end of the six-month study, the patients who had taken chondroitin sulfates had improved much more than those who had received the placebo (as measured by the Lequesne Index and VAS test of spontaneous joint pain). Another indication of improvement was the fact that those in the chondroitin sulfate group were able to walk a twenty-meter distance more rapidly than they had at the beginning of the study, but the placebo group could not. Finally, the chondroitin sulfate group needed less pain medicine than the placebo group. The researchers concluded that chondroitin sulfates behave as a "slow-acting drug" useful for treating osteoarthritis of the knee.

4. L. Busci et al., "Efficacy and Tolerability of 2×400 mg Oral Chondroitin Sulfate as a Single Dose in the Treatment of Knee Osteoarthritis."

Chondroitin Outperforms Placebo[5]

For reasons we don't yet fully understand, placebos (''sugar'' pills with no medicinal value) sometimes act like real medicines. Countless studies have shown that if you give placebos to patients suffering from a wide variety of ailments but tell them that it's ''real'' medicine, 30 percent or more will feel better as a result of the *placebo effect*. Thus, to make sure that a new medicine's results are the real thing and not the placebo effect, it is generally necessary to compare the new medicine to a placebo in a double-blind study where neither the patients nor the doctors know who is getting the real thing until the study has been completed.

A group of European researchers pitted chondroitin sulfates against a placebo in a three-month, randomized, double-blind, multicenter study of 127 patients suffering from osteoarthritis in one or both knees. Two different tests, the Lequesne Index and VAS (which measures spontaneous joint pain), were used to measure the degree of pain at the beginning and end of the study.

Forty-three of the participants were given 400 mg of chondroitin sulfates three times per day, forty patients were given 1,200 mg of chondroitin sulfates once per day, while forty-four received the placebo. Neither the doctors nor the patients knew who was taking the chondroitin sulfates and who the placebo until the final results were analyzed.

Results: The patients taking chondroitin sulfates enjoyed significant reduction of clinical symptoms as measured by the Lequesne Index and VAS compared with the placebo group. Interestingly, the patients taking chondroitin sulfates once per day did equally as well as those taking them three times per day.

5. P. Bourgeois, G. Chales, J. Dehais, B. Melcambre, P. Dreyfus, J.-L. Kuntz, and S. Rosenberg, ''Efficacy and Tolerability of Chondroitin Sulfate 1200 mg/day vs. Chondroitin Sulfate 3×400 mg/day vs. Placebo.''

Chondroitin Sulfates Stand the Test of Time[6]

One of the key factors one looks for in a medicine is its ability to continue working over time. This is important, for the body can become habituated to a substance—get so used to it that it's no longer effective. Indeed, many medicines can be used for only a short while before they lose effectiveness.

Chondroitin sulfates were put to the test of time in a year-long, randomized, double-blind, placebo-controlled study involving patients suffering from osteoarthritis of the knee. The test was randomized, which means that people were arbitrarily assigned to either the chondroitin or placebo groups. It was double-blind, so that neither the doctors nor the patients knew who was receiving which until the end.

At the end of the study, the twenty-five patients taking chondroitin sulfates and the twenty-two on placebo were tested and compared.

Results: Compared to the placebo group, the chondroitin group enjoyed significantly increased mobility in the affected joints as evaluated using the Lysholm score and significantly less joint swelling, instability, and effusion. In six of the twenty-five patients on chondroitin, the cartilage surface was smoother or thicker, a sign of increased cartilage health. There were no such improvements in the placebo group, and in three of the twenty-two of them, the affected cartilage looked thinner or more damaged. The placebo group also took significantly more paracetamol than those in the chondroitin group, indicating that chondroitin was blocking pain as well. Due to side effects, three patients dropped out during the study in the placebo group while none did in the treatment group. The researchers concluded that "chondroitin is a symptomatic slow

6. A. M. Fleisch, C. Merlin, A. Imhoff, J. Hodler, and R. Kissling, "A One-Year Randomized, Double-Blind, Placebo-Controlled Study with Oral Chondroitin Sulfate in Patients with Knee Osteoarthritis."

acting drug for the treatment of knee osteoarthritis with a good clinical outcome.''

Chondroitin Sulfate Stops Joint Degeneration[7]

In this study conducted jointly by American and French researchers, chondroitin sulfate was found to halt the progression of osteoarthritic joint degradation as determined by quantitative X-ray analysis. Forty-two men and women suffering from osteoarthritis of the knee, and ranging in age from thirty-five to seventy-eight, were given either 800 mg of chondroitin sulfate orally per day or a placebo. The participants were tested and radiographs were taken at the beginning of the study and a year later when the study concluded.

Results: The mean thickness of the femoro-tibial joint (in the knee) decreased significantly in those taking the placebo, while it held steady in those who received the chondroitin sulfates. The femoro-tibial joint surface area also decreased in the placebo group, but not in the chondroitin group. Impressed by these positive results, the researchers concluded that chondroitin sulfates have ''the characteristics of a chondromodulating and structural-modifying agent.'' In other words, chondroitin sulfates do more than relieve pain and swelling. They can actually halt the progress of osteoarthritis by making positive changes in the cartilage structure.

Glucosamine Modifies the Course of Osteoarthritis[8]

Italian researchers investigated glucosamine's ability to relieve the symptoms of osteoarthritis by giving either glucosamine,

7. D. Uebelhart, E. J. M. A. Thonar, P. D. Delmas, A. Chantraine, and E. Vignon, ''Chondroitin 4 & 6 Sulfate. A Symptomatic Slow-Acting Drug for Osteoarthritis, Does Also Have Structural Modifying Properties.''
8. L. C. Rovati, ''The Clinical Profile of Glucosamine Sulfate as a Selective Symptom Modifying Drug in Osteoarthritis: Current Data and Perspectives.''

a placebo, piroxicam, a standard NSAID, or a combination of glucosamine plus the piroxicam for a period of three months to 329 patients in a randomized, controlled, double-blind study. The Lequesne Index again was used as the assessment tool.

Results: Glucosamine was far more effective than either the placebo or NSAID during the study period. Also, the side effect profile was better in the glucosamine group than any of the others: Glucosamine, 14.8 percent; placebo, 23.7 percent; piroxicam, 40.9 percent; and the combination, 35.0 percent. Furthermore, whereas the NSAID's effectiveness wore off during the two-month follow-up period (despite being the longest-acting NSAID on the market), glucosamine continued to work, suggesting that not only does it block pain, but it does so by actually fixing at least part of the problem in the joint (and not simply by covering up pain, as standard medicines do).

Glucosamine Versus Ibuprofen[9]

This double-blind study involved 178 people suffering from osteoarthritis of the knee. During the four-week study period, the volunteers were given either 1,500 mg per day of glucosamine or 1,200 mg of ibuprofen, a standard NSAID.

Results: The glucosamine was as effective as ibuprofen for pain control but was "significantly better tolerated." Ten percent of the patients dropped out of the ibuprofen group due to adverse drug reactions, whereas none of the users of glucosamine sulfate dropped out. This means that the natural glucosamine did not have the side effects typically seen with NSAIDs, side effects that can discourage patients from taking their medicine, or may actually harm them.

9. G. X. Qiu, S. N. Gao, and I. Setnikar, "Efficacy and Safety of Glucosamine Sulfate vs. Ibuprofen in Patients with Knee Osteoarthritis."

Therapeutic Effect of a Mixture of Glucosamine Sulfate and Chondroitin[10]

A well-known method of producing an inflammatory type of arthritis (more like rheumatoid than osteoarthritis) is to inject a soluble form of type-II collagen right into the joints of animals. This study, using forty-five rats, was done at Johns Hopkins University. Twenty-four of the rats were given an oral mixture of glucosamine and chondroitin for ten days prior to, and thirty-two days after, joint injections with the soluble type-II collagen. Twenty-three rats were simply injected without the pretreatment.

Results: Twenty-two (96.5 percent) of the rats that did not receive the glucosamine and chondroitin developed arthritis (as determined by microscopic and chemical analysis). In the rats who did get treated, only thirteen (54 percent) developed arthritis! This was an impressive difference. Although this was an animal study, it certainly presents convincing evidence of the disease-modifying effects of glucosamine and chondroitin.

Overall, there has been much attention worldwide regarding the use of glucosamine and chondroitin for the treatment of arthritis. With the tremendously positive results that have been reported, there's no doubt that the trend toward greater use of these remarkable supplements will continue.

10. J. J. Beren, S. L. Hill, and N. R. Rose, "Therapeutic Effect of Cosamin® on Autoimmune Type II Collagen-Induced Arthritis in Rats."

Appendix B

Resources

American Academy of Osteopathy
3500 Depauw Boulevard
Suite 1080
Indianapolis, IN 46268-1136
317-879-1881

American Academy of Physical Medicine and Rehabilitation
122 South Michigan Avenue
Suite 1300
Chicago, IL 60603-6107
312-922-9366

American Chiropractic Association
1916 Wilson Boulevard
Suite 300
Arlington, VA 22201
703-276-8800

Arthritis Foundation
1330 W. Peachtree Street
Atlanta, GA 30309
404-872-7100
www.arthritis.org

Feldenkrais Guild
PO Box 11145
San Francisco, CA 94101
415-550-8708

International Yoga Institute
227 West 13th Street
New York, NY 10011
212-929-0586

Rolf Institute
PO Box 1868
Boulder, CO 80302
303-449-5903

Dr. Jason Theodosakis
6890 East Sunrise
#120-383
Tucson, AZ 85750

Brenda Adderly, M.H.A.
144 N. Robertson Blvd.
Suite 103
Los Angeles, CA 90048

On the Web

www.arthritis.org
The official site of the Arthritis Foundation